O A N L
OXFORD AMERICAN NEUROLOGY LIBRARY

Multiple Sclerosis

O A N L
OXFORD AMERICAN NEUROLOGY LIBRARY

Multiple Sclerosis

Clinician's Guide to Diagnosis and Treatment

Gary Birnbaum, MD

Director, Multiple Sclerosis Treatment and Research Center
Minneapolis Clinic of Neurology
Clinical Professor of Neurology
University of Minnesota School of Medicine
Minneapolis, MN

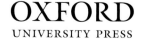

OXFORD
UNIVERSITY PRESS

OXFORD
UNIVERSITY PRESS

Oxford University Press, Inc., publishes works that further
Oxford University's objective of excellence
in research, scholarship, and education.

Oxford New York
Auckland Cape Town Dar es Salaam Hong Kong Karachi
Kuala Lumpur Madrid Melbourne Mexico City Nairobi
New Delhi Shanghai Taipei Toronto

With offices in
Argentina Austria Brazil Chile Czech Republic France Greece
Guatemala Hungary Italy Japan Poland Portugal Singapore
South Korea Switzerland Thailand Turkey Ukraine Vietnam

Copyright © 2009 by Oxford University Press, Inc.

Published by Oxford University Press, Inc.
198 Madison Avenue, New York, New York 10016
www.oup.com

Oxford is a registered trademark of Oxford University Press

Birnbaum, Gary.
Multiple sclerosis : clinician's guide to diagnosis and treatment / Gary Birnbaum.
p. ; cm. — (Oxford American neurology library)
Includes bibliographical references.
ISBN 978-0-19-537316-5 (standard ed.)
1. Multiple sclerosis.   I. Title.   II. Series.
[DNLM: 1. Multiple Sclerosis. WL 360 B619m 2008]
RC377.B56 2008
616.8'34–dc22   2008023814

9 8 7 6 5 4 3 2 1
Printed in USA
on acid-free paper

Acknowledgment

This book would not have been possible without my being privileged to care for the many persons with MS, in some instances over decades. They have taught me all I know about this disease. Their courage, resilience, and optimism in the face of an illness with potentially major consequences have been a continuing source of inspiration and support. I thank them for all they have given me.

Needless to say, my wife, daughter, and her family supported my efforts and indulged me the time away from them to write this book. I thank them too.

Finally, I thank Drs. Benjamin Baker and John Money, two of my professors at Johns Hopkins, who, unbeknownst to them, were role models to me of physicians who provided compassionate, understanding, gentle, and expert care to their patients, and made it look easy.

Gary Birnbaum, MD

Contents

Introduction

Many books have been written on the pathology, immunology, diagnosis, and treatment of persons with multiple sclerosis (MS). Most of these have been directed at neurologists and other specialists in the field, with details commensurate with the expertise of these readers. This book has a different purpose. Its goal is to present a practical and reasonable approach to the diagnosis and treatment of MS to those health professionals most likely to first see persons with MS, namely primary care physicians and clinical nurse specialists. The long-term care of persons with MS often is dependent on the expertise of such non-neurologists, but with the multitude of other illnesses cared for by primary care health professionals, providing a compendium of all known information about MS is not useful. Rather, I hope that this book will provide an algorithm for the diagnosis and treatment of persons with MS, as well as providing a foundation for more detailed readings on the subject.

As is quickly apparent at any meeting of MS "experts," there is no "one way" to manage persons with MS. The variability in disease presentation, disease course, and variety of symptoms mandates an individualized approach. The approaches to be described in this book are those I have found useful over more than 30 years of caring for persons with MS. I don't espouse them as being "the only way" but I hope they will serve as a framework for providing the best possible care to our patients.

Chapter 1

A Brief History of MS

It is not possible to define the historical onset of a disease characterized not only by a particular clinical course but also by particular changes in the central nervous system (CNS; brain and spinal cord), since the technology necessary to look at changes in the CNS was not available until the late 19th century. However, by interpreting biographies and diaries of persons with symptoms suggestive of MS, it is possible that MS occurred as early as the 14th century.

In a biography of St. Lidwina of Schiedam, symptoms suggestive of a fluctuating, multifocal neurologic illness are described that started in the year 1396 after ice skating. Her subsequent course of increased walking difficulties, with episodes that may have been remissions, suggests that she may have had MS, though this is far from certain. St. Lidwina was canonized in 1890 and is now the patron saint of skaters.

A more robust description of symptoms strongly suggestive of MS is found in the diary of Sir Augustus Frederick d'Este (1794–1848), a grandson of England's King George III. In it he describes exacerbating remitting symptoms suggestive of optic neuritis with double vision, leg weakness, and bowel and bladder difficulties, followed over the years by gradually progressive weakness and spasms that left him bed-bound by the end of his life.

Why is a history of MS put into a book that is meant to be a primer on the diagnosis and care of persons with MS? For two reasons. One is to put into historical context the fact that MS occurred before the appearance of many modern toxins that have been impugned as causes of MS. These include mercury amalgam in tooth fillings (first used in the early 20th century) and environmental lead. That does not mean that environmental factors are unimportant in MS: as will be described in Chapter 2, environmental factors play a major role in disease susceptibility. Rather, in the absence of proof implicating a particular factor, great caution should be used in recommending any "treatments" based on unsupported hypotheses, such as advising persons with MS to have their dental amalgams removed. The second reason for having this chapter is to put into historical context the fact that any treatment for a disease such as MS, which can spontaneously remit, will in some instances appear successful. Many of the treatments received by Sir d'Este, such as bloodletting, leeches to the temples, beefsteaks twice a day, sherry and Madeira wine, rubbing with horsehair gloves, and undergoing a course of electricity, were associated with significant improvement and certainly would have been considered successful therapies by the physicians of that time.

While MS was not recognized as a distinct disease until 20 years after d'Este's death, pathologic descriptions of diseased brain were being made with increasing frequency, and a professor of anatomy, Robert Carswell, in 1838 was the first to note patches of hardened areas of scarring in the brain and spinal cord of persons who now would be classified as having MS. However, there were no clinical correlations. Working independently, the anatomist Jean Cruveilhier (1791–1894), in a book published in 1841, described multifocal areas of scarring in the brain and spinal cord. Cruveilhier was the first person to correlate the pathologic changes with symptoms such as tremors and walking difficulties.

The Parisian neurologist Jean-Martin Charcot (1825–1893), with his colleague Edmé Vulpian, in a series of lectures in 1868 was instrumental in summarizing the observations of the anatomists and defining MS as a separate clinical disease. He also described both demyelination and axonal loss as characteristic pathologic features of the disease. It is said that Charcot saw fewer than 40 cases of MS in his lifetime, including his maid, whom he believed had this illness, and thus considered it rare. Nevertheless, his careful clinical and pathologic observations laid the foundation for much of the work on MS in the subsequent century.

Research into the epidemiology of MS around the world was accelerated by the efforts of the Association for Research in Nervous and Mental Diseases (ARNMD) in 1921, leading to the observations of Lord Russell Brain, who in 1930 was one of the first to describe the uneven geographic distribution of MS.

Experimental Autoimmune Encephalomyelitis

While MS is an exclusively human disease, much of our understanding of autoimmune phenomena in the CNS is based on an animal model initially called experimental allergic encephalomyelitis (EAE), induced by Thomas Rivers in 1935 following immunization of animals with CNS components. While there are major differences between MS and EAE, rodent EAE continues to be used as a model for MS and is used to establish "proof of concept" for potential treatments for MS. Indeed, all current therapies for MS were initially studied in EAE and were shown to be effective before being tested in humans. It is unlikely a therapy in this day and age would ever enter clinical trials without showing prior efficacy in ameliorating EAE. However, the majority of effective treatments of EAE have not proven to be effective when tested in human clinical trials.

EAE has also been useful in helping elucidate some of the presumed mechanisms of action of the disease-modifying therapies, described in Chapter 8. Since this book is intended to be a practical compilation of user-friendly data, a detailed description of changes in EAE induced by disease-modifying therapies is not indicated.

Further Reading

Brain WR. Critical review: disseminating sclerosis. *Q J Med*. 1930;23:343–391.

Carswell R. *Illustrations of the Elementary Forms of Disease*. London: Longman; 1838 (Plate 1V, Fig. 1).

Charcot JM. *Lectures on the diseases of the nervous system delivered at La Salpêtrière* (translated from French). London: The New Sydenham Society; 1877:170–177, 182–202.

Charcot JM. Histologie de la sclérose en plaques. *Gaz Hop (Paris)*. 1868;41:554, 557–558, 566.

Charcot M. *Lectures on Diseases of the Nervous System* (translated from French). London: The New Sydenham Society; 1881 (vol 1, p. 214).

Cruveilhier J. *L'Anatomie pathologique du corps humain; descriptions avec figures lithographiées et coloriées: diverses alterations morbides dont le corps humain est susceptible*. Paris: Baillière; 1829–1842 (vol 2; liv 32, Pl 2, pp. 19–24; liv 38, Pl 5, pp. 1–4).

Firth D. *The Case of Augustus D'Este*. Cambridge: Cambridge University Press; 1948.

Murray J. Prelude to the framing of a disease: multiple sclerosis in the period before Charcots Lecons. *Int Mult Scler J*. 2004;11(3):79–85.

Murray J. *Multiple Sclerosis—The History of a Disease*. New York: Demos Medical Publishing; 2005.

Chapter 2

Factors Involved in Causing Multiple Sclerosis

Epidemiology

Geographic Distribution

MS occurs worldwide, but its incidence varies greatly. MS is most common in temperate climates, both above and below the equator, with diminishing frequency as one approaches the equator. The reasons for this uneven distribution are not clear, but one important factor must be environmental exposure. There are major differences in exposures to viral, bacterial, and parasitic agents in different geographic areas, as well as differences in the ages at which individuals are exposed to these agents. Migration studies of populations moving from higher-risk to lower-risk regions, or vice versa, have convincingly shown that living in a particular risk area before puberty establishes the risk for that individual; moving subsequently does not change the risk. Thus, an early environmental event, possibly infectious, is important in determining susceptibility to disease. Many factors have been implicated; among them are exposure to Epstein-Barr virus and exposure to, or lack of exposure to, sunlight and vitamin D.

Of particular concern are the recent observations that the incidence of MS has doubled in the past century, almost exclusively in women, with little change in the incidence of MS in men. These differences are not just due to better ascertainment of disease, since the rise in incidence was noted very early in the 20th century, before the advent of magnetic resonance imaging (MRI) or newer laboratory techniques. While the reasons for these changes are not known, it is known that the advent of the industrial revolution resulted in major changes in environment as well as in health care. Discerning which factors are important in initiating the disease remains a major challenge, since the environmental factor responsible may long be gone or unremembered by the time a person with MS is diagnosed with the disease. Populations that may allow ascertainment of important environmental factors are children and adolescents with MS. Because of their very early onset of disease, they may be chronologically closer to the triggering event than adults (see Chapter 11).

Gender

As a group, MS is more common in women than in men. The differences are most pronounced in persons with the relapsing-remitting form of MS and least pronounced in persons with the primary-progressive form of MS (see Chapter 3). In relapsing-remitting MS, the ratio of women to men is about 2 to 3:1. Such differences suggest that genetic and hormonal factors play a key role in defining susceptibility, especially genes on the X and Y chromosomes. In support of this conjecture is the observation that MS becomes relatively quiescent during pregnancy, only to reappear with increased frequency after delivery. In primary-progressive MS, a form of disease occurring in older individuals, the ratio of females to males approaches 1:1. Characteristics of the different patterns of MS are described in Chapter 3.

Age

In general, MS presents in the second to sixth decade of life. MS can occur in prepubertal children and can present after age 60, but such instances are unusual. This raises the possibility that the pathogenesis of disease in persons at the extremes of age may be different. As will be discussed in Chapter 4, the biologic changes of MS, as seen on MRI, can occur many years before the clinical presentation, owing to the ability of the brain to compensate for areas of milder injury. Indeed, there are reports of persons who, at autopsy, had classic pathologic changes of MS but had no clinical symptoms.

Studies have been done trying to correlate the age of clinical onset of disease with severity. Some have suggested that a later age of onset is associated with more severe disease, but this is not uniformly found. An early age of onset is associated with a slower clinical course, but the age to reach a particular level of disability is earlier.

Race

MS is most common in persons of Northern European extraction. It can occur in other groups of individuals but often, as is the case with African Americans, there are ancestors from Northern Europe. A variant of MS occurs in persons of Asian background. It involves mainly the eyes and spinal cord and is called opticospinal MS, neuromyelitis optica, or Devic's disease. Differences between this form of MS and forms of MS in non-Asians are described in Chapter 3.

Some ethnic groups are relatively resistant to developing MS. These include Native American Indians, the Inuit, and African blacks. In addition, relatively segregated ethnic groups, such as the Hutterites, also are resistant to MS, even though they live in high-risk geographic areas. These observations provide strong evidence for the role of genes in determining susceptibility to MS, despite exposure to environments that increase disease risk.

Causes of MS

The cause of MS is not known. As described in Chapter 3, MS may be a syndrome and not a disease, with different pathogenic pathways leading to CNS demyelination and axonal loss. Nevertheless, there are several tenable hypotheses that could explain the development of this disease.

Genes

There are strong data indicating a major role for genes in determining susceptibility to MS. Most important are family studies showing that 25% of individuals with MS have another family member, up to the first-cousin level, with this disease. Twin studies also show that the concordance rate for MS among identical twins can be as high as 30% to 40%, with lesser but still higher-than-expected rates in non-identical twins and other siblings.

In addition, genetic typing studies show that particular genes of the major histocompatibility complex (MHC genes) are associated with the development of disease, especially the class II genes. The genotype most noted in Northern Europeans is DR15-DQ6, with different class II genes associated with MS in Southern Europeans. The common thread is that class II MHC genes play a major role in immune system functioning, supporting the hypothesis that MS is associated with a particular pattern of immune responses, possibly to environmental antigens. These, in turn, lead to CNS tissue destruction. Genes of the MHC account for up to 40% of the genetic factors involved in disease susceptibility. Of interest are recent observations that males appear to transmit susceptibility to MS more than females. Also of interest are the observations that patterns of MS vary among family members with the disease: some will have relapsing-remitting MS, some primary-progressive MS, and some "biologic MS" (that is, changes on MRI and in spinal fluid suggestive of MS but without any clinical manifestations).[1,2] Identifying the reasons for such differences will provide important insights into the role of genes in determining susceptibility.

More recent studies have involved screening the entire human genome for changes in single nucleotides (called single nucleotide polymorphisms [SNPs]). These large, multicenter studies revealed an increase in a particular SNP in the gene coding for the receptor for the immunologic cytokine, IL-7. This particular SNP is also found in a large number of normal individuals; thus, having this nucleotide substitution accounts for only 2% of the genetic susceptibility to MS.

One can conclude from these studies that there is no single "MS gene" involved in susceptibility; and possibly dozens of genes are determinate. It is almost certain that genes will also be involved in determining the severity of disease, pattern of disease, and responses to disease-modifying therapies. The latter group of genes will be of particular importance in choosing appropriate therapies for persons with MS.

Environmental Factors

Based on the geographic distribution of MS, environmental factors play a significant role in determining susceptibility to MS. The nature of such factors is not known, but data suggest that an infectious agent may play a role.

Exposure to infectious agents varies with latitude. Persons in tropical regions are exposed to very different bacterial, viral, and parasitic agents than are persons in temperate zones. In addition, the age of exposure may also be a critical variable, since the pattern of response to an infectious agent varies with the maturity of the individual's immune system. This is best exemplified by the patterns of response seen to polio virus: early exposure to virus results only in an enteric illness, whereas exposure later in life increases the risk of paralytic disease.

Many infectious agents have been implicated in the pathogenesis of MS. These include chlamydia, measles virus, herpes simplex type 6, Epstein-Barr virus, and varicella. The issue is complicated by the fact that persons with active MS have a generalized activation of immune cells with increased amounts of antibodies to multiple antigens, including viral antigens. Nevertheless, several recent studies suggest that early exposure to the Epstein-Barr virus is one susceptibility factor for the development of MS.

Additional support for a role of infection in initiating MS is provided by the observations of John Kurtzke and colleagues. They identified an epidemic of MS in the Faroe Islands, an isolated cluster of islands off the coast of Denmark, which occurred after the islands were occupied during World War II by "foreign" British soldiers. Before that time MS was unknown among Faroe Island inhabitants. Several years after the British arrived, a flurry of persons with MS were identified, with another flurry about 10 years after the first. Attempts to identify the environmental, possibly infectious, agent involved were unsuccessful.

As noted previously, the incidence of MS in women has more than doubled in the past century, a phenomenon not noted in men. The industrial and scientific revolutions resulted in large numbers of changes in both the environment and in health care, such as improved sanitary facilities (e.g., indoor plumbing and toilets), early childhood vaccinations, and changes in air quality and temperature. How these relate to MS susceptibility is not known, nor do they explain the gender-specific rise in incidence among women. One possibility is that with the industrial revolution and the changes in air quality, the amount of exposure to sunlight and ultraviolet light has decreased, resulting in decreased levels of vitamin D, a vitamin produced in the skin by exposure to sunlight. Retrospective studies of persons with MS have shown that such individuals had decreased levels of vitamin D before the onset of their illness compared to persons who did not develop the disease. Whether vitamin D is a marker for other factors involved in susceptibility or is itself etiologically important is not known. What *is* known is that vitamin D plays an important role in maintaining normal functioning of the immune system and thus could be both etiologically significant and a potential treatment for the disease. Studies in this regard are under way.

Immunology

Volumes have been written on the immunologic changes associated with MS, and it is beyond the scope of this tome to detail these changes. Suffice it to say that MS is believed to be an autoimmune disease, one in which there is a loss of immune tolerance to CNS antigens. As a result, an individual with the "proper" susceptibility genes, exposed to an as-yet-undefined environmental factor, mounts an immune response to CNS tissues. The requirement for such a confluence of factors is supported by the fact that almost all humans have within their "immune repertoire" cells that can be sensitized to CNS proteins. Thus, under certain conditions, such as immunization with CNS tissues, persons can develop the capacity to immunologically attack their brain.[3,4] The immune system itself is normal in persons with MS, though they have a slightly higher incidence of other autoimmune diseases such as thyroid disease and inflammatory bowel disease. What remains controversial is whether MS results from an "inside-out" CNS abnormality or CNS destruction occurs as a result of an "outside-in" change.

Proponents of the "inside-out" hypothesis suggest that the primary event in MS occurs within the CNS and involves the destruction and degeneration of oligodendrocytes, the myelin-producing cells. A leading advocate of this is John Prineas, who, along with colleagues, has described noninflammatory degeneration of oligodendrocytes in persons very early in the course of their disease.[5] He proposes that this destruction of oligodendrocytes, of unknown cause, leads to a release of formerly sequestered antigens into the periphery, resulting in sensitization of the immune system, loss of immune tolerance to CNS proteins, and subsequent immune-mediated tissue injury.

Proponents of the "outside-in" hypothesis propose that the initiating event in MS is a breakdown of immune tolerance to CNS proteins due to an environmental factor, possibly infectious. The immune response to the infectious agent results in a cross-reactive immune response to CNS antigens and an attack on brain tissue leading to tissue injury.

Which of these hypotheses is correct is not known. What *is* known, as will be discussed in Chapter 3, is that immune-mediated CNS inflammation plays a critical role in disease pathogenesis, and that controlling such inflammation with disease-modifying therapies (discussed in Chapter 8) alters the course of the disease.

Multiple mechanisms of immune-mediated tissue destruction have been described. The most popular one at this time is that CNS-sensitized lymphocytes enter the brain following adherence to brain capillary endothelium, are then restimulated by tissue antigens, and as a result release toxic substances, such as cytokines, resulting in demyelination and axonal loss. Toxic cytokines include IL-17, interferon-gamma, and tumor necrosis factor. New data also suggest that B cells have an important role to play in MS pathogenesis, either in their capacity to produce toxic antibodies or in their abilities to present antigens to toxic T cells. Once inflammation occurs in the CNS, resident macrophages, called microglia, become activated, and these too then produce toxic substances, such as nitric oxide, that result in tissue injury.

Given the multiplicity of immunologic events occurring as a result of loss of CNS tolerance, multiple attempts at intervention in this cascade have been made. Some have been successful, but most have not, with some even resulting in worsening of disease. The reader is referred to more extensive reviews on the immunologic changes in MS noted below.[6–8]

References

1. Hensiek AE, Seaman SR, Barcellos LF, et al. Familial effects on the clinical course of multiple sclerosis. *Neurology*. 2007;68(5):376–383.

2. Hupperts R, Broadley S, Mander A, et al. Patterns of disease in concordant parent-child pairs with multiple sclerosis. *Neurology*. 2001;57(2):290–295.

3. Neurological Clinical Pathological Conference: Encephalomyelitis due to rabies vaccine (bulbospinal type); massive pulmonary embolism. *Dis Nerv Syst*. 1950;11(10):310–316.

4. Pathak R, Khare KC. Disseminated sclerosis syndrome following antirabic vaccination. *J Indian Med Assoc*. 1967;49(10):484–485.

5. Barnett MH, Prineas JW. Relapsing and remitting multiple sclerosis: pathology of the newly forming lesion. *Ann Neurol*. 2004;55(4):458–468.

6. Anderton SM, Liblau RS. Regulatory T cells in the control of inflammatory demyelinating diseases of the central nervous system. *Curr Opin Neurol*. 2008;21(3):248–254.

7. Holmoy T, Hestvik AL. Multiple sclerosis: immunopathogenesis and controversies in defining the cause. *Curr Opin Infect Dis*. 2008;21(3):271–278.

8. Bar-Or A. The immunology of multiple sclerosis. *Semin Neurol*. 2008;28(1):29–45.

Further Reading

Alonso A, Jick SS, Olek MJ, et al. Incidence of multiple sclerosis in the United Kingdom: findings from a population-based cohort. *J Neurol*. 2007; 254(12):1736–1741.

Ascherio A, Munger KL. Environmental risk factors for multiple sclerosis. Part I: The role of infection. *Ann Neurol*. 2007;61(4):288–299.

Ascherio A, Munger KL. Environmental risk factors for multiple sclerosis. Part II: Noninfectious factors. *Ann Neurol*. 2007;61(6):504–513.

Debouverie M, Pitton-Vouyovitch S, Louis S, et al. Increasing incidence of multiple sclerosis among women in Lorraine, Eastern France. *Mult Scler*. 2007;13(8):962–967.

Ebers GC. Environmental factors and multiple sclerosis. *Lancet Neurol*. 2008;7(3):268–277.

Gregory SG, Schmidt S, Seth P, et al. Interleukin 7 receptor alpha chain (IL7R) shows allelic and functional association with multiple sclerosis. *Nat Genet*. 2007;39(9):1083–1091.

Grimaldi LM, Palmeri B, Salemi G, et al. High prevalence and fast-rising incidence of multiple sclerosis in Caltanissetta, Sicily, southern Italy. *Neuroepidemiology*. 2007;28(1):28–32.

Hafler DA, Compston A, Sawcer S, et al. Risk alleles for multiple sclerosis identified by a genome-wide study. *N Engl J Med*. 2007;357(9):851–862.

Hernan MA, Olek MJ, Ascherio A. Geographic variation of MS incidence in two prospective studies of US women. *Neurology*. 1999;53(8):1711–1718.

Holick MF. Vitamin D deficiency. *N Engl J Med*. 2007;357(3):266–281.

Kantarci OH, Barcellos LF, Atkinson EJ, et al. Men transmit MS more often to their children vs women: the Carter effect. *Neurology*. 2006;67(2):305–310.

Kurtzke JF. Multiple sclerosis in time and space—geographic clues to cause. *J Neurovirol*. 2000;6(Suppl 2):S134–140.

Kurtzke JF, Heltberg A. Multiple sclerosis in the Faroe Islands: an epitome. *J Clin Epidemiol.* 2001;54(1):1–22.

Kurtzke JF, Hyllested K. Multiple sclerosis in the Faroe Islands: I. Clinical and epidemiological features. *Ann Neurol.* 1979;5(1):6–21.

Kurtzke JF, Hyllested K. Multiple sclerosis in the Faroe Islands. II. Clinical update, transmission, and the nature of MS. *Neurology.* 1986;36(3):307–328.

Lipton HL, Liang Z, Hertzler S, et al. A specific viral cause of multiple sclerosis: one virus, one disease. *Ann Neurol.* 2007;61(6):514–523.

Marrie RA. Environmental risk factors in multiple sclerosis aetiology. *Lancet Neurol.* 2004;3(12):709–718.

Munger KL, Levin LI, Hollis BW, et al. Serum 25-hydroxyvitamin D levels and risk of multiple sclerosis. *JAMA.* 2006;296(23):2832–2838.

Nielsen TR, Pedersen M, Rostgaard K, et al. Correlations between Epstein-Barr virus antibody levels and risk factors for multiple sclerosis in healthy individuals. *Mult Scler.* 2007;13(3):420–423.

Niino M, Fukuzawa T, Kikuchi S, et al. Therapeutic potential of vitamin D for multiple sclerosis. *Curr Med Chem.* 2008;15(5):499–505.

Orton SM, Herrera BM, Yee IM, et al. Sex ratio of multiple sclerosis in Canada: a longitudinal study. *Lancet Neurol.* 2006;5(11):932–936.

Poser CM. The dissemination of multiple sclerosis: a Viking saga? A historical essay. *Ann Neurol.* 1994;36(Suppl 2):S231–243.

Smolders J, Damoiseaux J, Menheere P, et al. Vitamin D as an immune modulator in multiple sclerosis, a review. *J Neuroimmunol.* 2008;194(1–2):7–17.

Tienari P, Bonetti A, Pinlaja H, et al. Multiple sclerosis in G: genes and geography. *Clin Neurol Neurosurg.* 2006;108(3):223–226.

Willer CJ, Dyment DA, Risch NJ, et al. Twin concordance and sibling recurrence rates in multiple sclerosis. *Proc Natl Acad Sci USA.* 2003;100(22):12877–12882.

Chapter 3

The Patterns and Pathophysiology of MS

Patterns of MS

The only invariable thing that can be said about the course of MS is that it is variable. There are, however, certain general patterns of disease that must be identified, since they imply certain pathophysiologic processes and indicate the use of particular disease-modifying therapies. Patterns of disease are based almost exclusively on the recollections of the individual with MS and the skills of the neurologic examiner. Thus, the following categories are not crisp and clean and often overlap. The clinical patterns of MS tell only part of the story in terms of identifying disease activity. As will be discussed in Chapter 4, disease processes, with associated tissue destruction, often are clinically silent. Thus, individuals may appear to be doing well clinically at a particular point, yet their disease may still be biologically active, increasing the chances of subsequent disability.

Relapsing-Remitting MS

The most common clinical pattern in persons with MS is one of relapsing-remitting, or partially remitting, episodes of neurologic dysfunction. The onset of neurologic changes can be rapid, appearing over several hours, or more indolent, appearing over days to weeks. Often the onset is focal and then spreads to involve additional body regions.

Symptoms and signs may persist for days, weeks, and even months, then resolve to varying degrees. Early in the disease relapses can resolve completely, but as the disease progresses, recovery to baseline becomes less common. Changes that persist at the end of a year usually are permanent. The frequency of attacks varies considerably, and this has important implications for prognosis. Long intervals between attacks and good recoveries from attacks are better prognostic indicators. Persons with relapsing-remitting MS are usually younger at onset; are predominantly women; and respond well to both acute anti-inflammatory treatments, such as steroids, and long-term immune-modulating therapies.

Determining an attack, relapse, or exacerbation can be difficult since many secondary variables can increase neurologic symptoms in MS. These include infections, fevers, heat, and fatigue. Changes in neurologic function brought on by superimposed body stressors are considered "pseudo-exacerbations" and are not indicative of new, inflammatory CNS processes. Rather, they result from decompensation of existing CNS scars and thus do not require treatment with anti-inflammatory drugs. Relapses and their management will be discussed in Chapter 7.

Benign MS and Biologic MS

To an extent, the term "benign MS" is an oxymoron. Even if an individual's illness is mild and not disabling, the psychological repercussions of the diagnosis can be significant. Yet within these constraints are persons with clinically definite MS who have no disability from their CNS disease.[1] Unfortunately, there are no established markers to identify such individuals prospectively, making the diagnosis of "benign MS" a retrospective one. Indeed, the longer one follows persons with MS, the smaller the number of individuals with a truly benign course.[2,3] The inability to predict the clinical course in persons with MS has important implications (see Chapter 8) in terms of initiation of disease-modifying therapies.

"Biologic MS" refers to individuals who have changes on CNS MRIs and in spinal fluid compatible with a multifocal CNS inflammatory process such as MS, but who are asymptomatic. First-degree relatives of MS patients, especially those with a family history of the disease, are often in this category. However, most neurologists have seen patients who have had MRIs for purposes other than diagnosing MS who have had lesions suggestive of this illness. Such individuals may remain asymptomatic all their lives, and treatment of persons with biologic MS is not indicated until clinical consequences of these lesions are manifest.

Secondary-Progressive MS

About half of the individuals with relapsing-remitting MS have a change in the pattern of their disease over time. The frequency of attacks or relapses decreases and eventually stops, only to be followed by a more insidious, gradual progression of their disabilities. This phase of their disease, progression without relapses, is called secondary-progressive MS. The transition between relapsing-remitting MS and secondary-progressive MS can be rapid or gradual, with no biologic marker to clearly separate the two. Persons with progressive symptoms yet with occasional relapses can be classified as having "transitional" disease, on their way to having more well-defined secondary-progressive MS. Persons in the secondary-progressive phase of illness have less acute inflammatory changes on their MRIs, such as new T2/FLAIR lesions or lesions with contrast enhancement. Rather, the lesion load noted on MRI may stabilize or actually decrease as cerebral atrophy becomes more prominent. Since acute inflammatory changes are not as prominent in secondary-progressive MS, anti-inflammatory drugs, such as steroids, are much less effective. Long-term immune-modulating therapies, to be discussed in Chapter 8, also are not effective.

Primary-Progressive MS

A neurologic wag once said, "Persons with primary-progressive MS are those who just can't remember their first relapse." This aphorism most likely is incorrect. In contrast to persons with relapsing-remitting MS, persons with primary-progressive MS cannot tell you a specific date of onset of symptoms. Rather, the symptoms appear gradually, over months to years, although their intensity may vary with fatigue, hot weather, or infections. Relapses, or acute changes in neurologic function, do not, by definition, precede the onset of neurologic difficulties. The course of disease varies greatly: some individuals have significant disability within 1 to 2 years, while in others progression is indolent, over decades. As a group, individuals with primary-progressive MS are older at disease onset, often in their 40s to 60, with a gender distribution of 50:50. The most common symptoms at onset reflect spinal cord dysfunction.[4–6] Most commonly there is a progressive lower extremity weakness, unilateral or bilateral, with or without numbness and tingling. In addition, changes in bowel, bladder, and sexual function are common. Less common symptoms at onset are cognitive changes and cerebellar symptoms, such as ataxia and limb incoordination. The pathophysiology of primary-progressive MS is different from that of relapsing-remitting MS, though some individuals have considerable overlap.[5,6]

Progressive-Relapsing MS

As noted previously, the patterns of disease in MS are defined almost exclusively by clinical parameters, either reported or observed.[7] Thus, it is not unexpected that some individuals meeting the criteria for primary-progressive MS at onset may, nevertheless, have superimposed relapses. General criteria for primary-progressive MS still apply, but persons with progressive-relapsing MS have more acute inflammatory activity in their CNS, and relapses can respond to treatment with short-term anti-inflammatory therapies. The value of long-term immune-modulating therapies is uncertain at this time.

Neuromyelitis Optica or Devic's Disease

Neuromyelitis optica (NMO) is an inflammatory, demyelinating CNS disease, different from MS in its pathophysiology, clinical course, and treatment.[8,9] It is included in this chapter as there can be overlaps between "classic" MS and NMO. NMO is much more common in persons of Asian extraction; it has a female preponderance and its course is characterized by acute episodes of optic neuritis, transverse myelitis, or a combination of the two. Intervals between episodes vary greatly, as do levels of impairment: many individuals have severe disability, mainly due to spinal cord dysfunction. Diagnosis is made on the basis of the clinical pattern, on radiologic grounds, with patients having relatively normal brain MRIs but long spinal cord T2/FLAIR lesions, extending over three or more segments. The cerebrospinal fluid often is without oligoclonal bands (see Chapter 5), and a blood test for the presence of antibodies to the CNS protein aquaporin 4 has recently been described that is relatively specific for NMO.[8] However, as more individuals are tested for the presence of antibodies to aquaporin 4 (NMO-IgG), it appears there are many gradations of NMO, with overlaps that may be indistinguishable from relapsing-remitting MS. The treatment of NMO is different from that of relapsing-remitting MS and is discussed in Chapter 7.

Table 3.1 Patterns of Disease

Disease Pattern	Distinguishing Features
Relapsing-remitting MS	1. Acute or subacute onset of neurologic symptoms and signs, lasting for days to months to years, with varying degrees of recovery. Attacks must be distinguished from "pseudo-exacerbations" occurring in a context of fever, infection, or fatigue. 2. Age of onset usually is 18 to 50 years of age, with a female preponderance. 3. CNS MRIs show varying numbers of lesions, both acute and chronic, in a pattern characteristic of MS (see Chapter 4), with increasing lesion load over time. 4. CSF shows changes of a low-grade inflammation (see Chapter 5).
Secondary-progressive MS	1. A history of relapsing-remitting symptoms and signs early in the disease, followed by a gradual progression of symptoms, at times with a transitional phase in which symptoms gradually progress, with an occasional relapse. 2. Age of onset is about 10 to 20 years after initial presentation of MS. 3. CNS MRIs show lesions of MS, but with few if any acute lesions, and progressive atrophy, and either gradually accumulating chronic lesions or a decline in lesion load as brain atrophy increases.
Primary-progressive MS	1. Gradual onset, over months to years, of neurologic symptoms and signs, most often resulting from spinal cord dysfunction. Occasionally there may be a relapse. 2. Age of onset usually later than relapsing-remitting MS, between 40 and 60 years. Equal male:female ratio. 3. CNS MRIs show lesions characteristic of MS, but often with a preponderance of lesions in the spinal cord. Usually lesions are chronic, but some individuals have numbers of acute lesions with contrast enhancement. 4. CSF shows signs of mild inflammation with or without the presence of oligoclonal bands.
Neuromyelitis optica	1. Rapid onset, over days, of optic nerve dysfunction, either unilateral or bilateral, and/or spinal cord dysfunction, usually in the form of a transverse myelitis 2. Age of onset is 20 to 40 years, with a female preponderance. 3. In a "classic" case, brain MRI is normal, with multisegment T2/FLAIR lesions of the spinal cord, but some patients have brain lesions. 4. CSF shows signs of mild to moderate inflammation but in the "classic" case will not have oligoclonal bands.

Pathophysiology of MS

There are increasing data showing that there are two separate, but probably interdependent, disease processes occurring in the CNS of persons with MS: acute inflammation and more indolent, chronic, low-grade inflammation and degeneration. Which comes first, and what are the initiating events? These remain unknown and are the subject of much controversy and speculation. Unfortunately, by the time a person presents with his or her first neurologic symptom, the initiating event(s) is long past, and disease processes may already be advanced. Retrieving these critical data will be essential to prevent and possibly cure the disease.

Acute Inflammation

A pathologic hallmark of MS is perivenular inflammation in white matter throughout the CNS, with infiltration of the surrounding tissues by a panoply of inflammatory cells, mainly multiple subpopulations of lymphocytes and mononuclear cells. Details of the complex immunology of these perivenular infiltrates is beyond the scope of this text. Suffice it to say that these cells are activated or "turned-on" inflammatory cells that secrete large numbers of biologically active substances, such as cytokines, chemokines, nitric oxide, and excitatory amino acids. These substances are toxic to the tissues of the brain, in particular myelin and axons. Adding to tissue injury are brain-antigen–specific T lymphocytes and non-antigen–specific macrophages that directly attack myelin. The results are varying degrees of myelin loss (demyelination) associated with alterations in the abilities of the underlying axons to relay electrical impulses. The resulting myelin loss exposes the "naked" axons to this toxic, inflammatory environment, and they too are transected and destroyed. Oligodendrocytes, the myelin-producing cells, are also killed, resulting in not only areas of intense tissue destruction but also regions with limited ability to regenerate and repair themselves. The intensity of inflammation varies among individuals; this may be one of the genetically defined variables of the disease. Severe inflammatory changes are associated with major axonal loss and are seen as "black holes," or hypointensities, on T1-weighted MRI imaging. Areas of new inflammation result in capillary damage, with breakdown of the blood–brain barrier. These areas can be seen on MRI as contrast-enhancing lesions (see Chapter 4).

Data suggest that different individuals have different pathogenic pathways resulting in acute myelin loss.[10] While these observations are still not universally accepted, they support the conjecture that MS may be a syndrome, with different processes leading to tissue destruction. A corollary of these observations would be that the effectiveness of therapies will vary among individuals with MS, depending on their disease phenotype. Preliminary observations support this conclusion.

While the most visible acute inflammation occurs in CNS white matter, recent observations show that inflammation also occurs in gray matter, both in cortex and in deep gray matter nuclei such as the thalamus. This inflammation appears to be different from that seen in white matter, with more B cells or antibody-producing cells present, and, at times, an accumulation of lymphocytes in patterns suggestive of lymphoid germinal centers.[11] These data suggest that different pathophysiologic processes are occurring concomitantly and may lead to different clinical outcomes. Cortical inflammation appears to be associated with more gray matter atrophy and more cognitive impairment, whereas inflammation in the deep cerebral tissues, brainstem, and spinal cord can lead to more impairment of motor, cerebellar, and sensory dysfunction.

Only one in ten lesions noted on MRI results in clinical symptoms. There may be several reasons for this. One may be related to the intensity of the tissue inflammation and the degree of tissue destruction. Perhaps more importantly, early in the disease there is sufficient plasticity in an individual's CNS to compensate for lesions that are in noncritical, or non-eloquent, areas. Plasticity may be lost with disease progression, resulting in less recovery between relapses and increasing disability.

The frequency of acute inflammation in MS varies considerably. In persons with very active disease, new lesions can occur almost constantly. In more indolent disease, new lesions, observable on MRI, can occur months to years apart and, as noted above, can be clinically silent. This fact has important clinical implications. Since much of MS disease activity can occur subclinically, in the absence of either relapses or changes on neurologic examination, monitoring of subclinical disease with MRI scanning is essential to determine the pattern of an individual's disease and his or her response to therapy. While there may be an "acute" disconnect between MRI changes and the clinical appearance of MS, data support the concept that increasing CNS damage, in particular atrophy and the appearance of "black holes," indicating axonal destruction, is associated over the long term with increasing disability.[2]

Chronic Inflammation and Degeneration

Charcot and others (see Chapter 1) noted even in the mid-19th century that MS was not only a demyelinating disease but also one associated with axonal destruction. Recent data not only support this observation but also indicate that low-grade, chronic, indolent inflammation is occurring throughout the CNS, resulting in loss of tissue and atrophy. Such changes are seen histologically in both white matter that appears normal on MRI and in gray matter. Indeed, using nonconventional MRI techniques, such as magnetization transfer (see Chapter 4) and brain volume measurement, brains in patients with MS are significantly different compared to control brains, with widespread decreases in tissue integrity and significantly greater rates of brain atrophy. These changes appear to be separate from the changes of acute inflammation, again suggesting that multiple pathogenic processes are occurring concurrently.

The histopathology of this chronic inflammation and degeneration is very different from that of acute inflammation. It results primarily from the diffuse infiltration of both gray and white matter by activated macrophages or microglia (resident macrophages in the CNS). These activated cells secrete many toxic substances, including cytokines and nitric oxide, and also have been shown to directly attack myelin, stripping it off axons.[12,13] In addition, there are diffuse increases in numbers of lymphocytes, mainly cytotoxic (CD8+) T cells in brains of patients with MS. Many of these cells are expanded from single cells (clones) and may be the result of a continuing recruitment of brain-specific immune cells into the CNS. Not known is whether the infiltrating T cells cause macrophage activation or whether they enter the CNS subsequent to macrophage activation.

In view of the multifaceted pathogenic processes that occur in the CNS in MS, combinations of anti-inflammatory and antidegenerative treatments may be needed to control this illness more completely.

Pathology of Neuromyelitis Optica

NMO, while originally classified as a variant of MS, appears to be a different disease. As noted above, many persons with NMO have antibodies to aquaporin 4. In addition, in contrast to MS, there are many B cells and high concentrations of antibodies and complement in the lesions of NMO, with extensive tissue necrosis in some individuals. As will be described in Chapter 7, this different pathologic process necessitates a different treatment approach.

References

1. Sayao AL, Devonshire V, Tremlett H. Longitudinal follow-up of "benign" multiple sclerosis at 20 years. *Neurology*. 2007;68:496–500.

2. Fisniku LK, Brex PA, Altmann DR et al. Disability and T2 MRI lesions: a 20-year follow-up of patients with relapse onset of multiple sclerosis. *Brain*. 2008;131:808–817.

3. Hirst CL, Ingram G, Swingler R, et al. Change in disability in patients with multiple sclerosis: A 20-year prospective population-based analysis. *J Neurol Neurosurg Psychiatry*. 2008 Feb. 26 [E-pub ahead of print].

4. Miller DH, Leary SM. Primary-progressive multiple sclerosis. *Lancet Neurol*. 2007;6:903–912.

5. Bruck W, Lucchinetti C, Lassmann H. The pathology of primary progressive multiple sclerosis. *Mult Scler*. 2002;8:93–97.

6. Lucchinetti C, Bruck W. The pathology of primary progressive multiple sclerosis. *Mult Scler*. 2004;10(Suppl 1):S23–30.

7. Lublin FD, Reingold SC. Defining the clinical course of multiple sclerosis: results of an international survey. National Multiple Sclerosis Society (USA) Advisory Committee on Clinical Trials of New Agents in Multiple Sclerosis. *Neurology*. 1996;46:907–911.

8. Weinshenker BG, Wingerchuk DM. Neuromyelitis optica: clinical syndrome and the NMO-IgG autoantibody marker. *Curr Top Microbiol Immunol*. 2008;318:343–356.

9. Wingerchuk DM, Lennon VA, Lucchinetti CF et al. The spectrum of neuromyelitis optica. *Lancet Neurol*. 2007;6:805–815.

10. Lucchinetti CF, Bruck W, Lassmann H. Evidence for pathogenic heterogeneity in multiple sclerosis. *Ann Neurol*. 2004;56:308.

11. Magliozzi R, Howell O, Vora A, et al. Meningeal B-cell follicles in secondary progressive multiple sclerosis associated with early onset of disease and severe cortical pathology. *Brain*. 2007;130:1089–1104.

12. Barnett MH, Henderson AP, Prineas JW. The macrophage in MS: just a scavenger after all? Pathology and pathogenesis of the acute MS lesion. *Mult Scler*. 2006;12:121–132.

13. Prineas JW, Kwon EE, Cho ES, et al. Immunopathology of secondary-progressive multiple sclerosis. *Ann Neurol*. 2001;50:646–657.

Further Reading

Brinar VV. Diagnostic and therapeutic dilemmas. *Clin Neurol Neurosurg.* 2004;106:180–186.

De Stefano N, Cocco E, Lai M, et al. Imaging brain damage in first-degree relatives of sporadic and familial multiple sclerosis. *Ann Neurol.* 2006;59:634–639.

Ge Y, Gonen O, Inglese M, et al. Neuronal cell injury precedes brain atrophy in multiple sclerosis. *Neurology.* 2004;62(4):624–627.

Morioka C, Komatsu Y, Tsujio T, et al. The evolution of the concentric lesions of atypical multiple sclerosis on MRI. *Radiat Med.* 1994;12(3):129–133.

Siva A. The spectrum of multiple sclerosis and treatment decisions. *Clin Neurol Neurosurg.* 2006;108:333–338.

Stuve O, Bennett JL, Hemmer B, et al. Pharmacological treatment of early multiple sclerosis. *Drugs.* 2008;68:73–83.

Chapter 4

Imaging of the Central Nervous System in Multiple Sclerosis

The diagnosis of MS is made almost exclusively on clinical grounds (see Chapter 5). There are no laboratory tests uniquely abnormal in MS, and using a test result to make such a diagnosis can lead to serious errors. However, laboratory tests, in particular imaging of the CNS, if interpreted in the context of the clinical picture, play an important role not only in supporting a diagnosis of MS but also in helping to determine a person's response to disease-modifying therapy. Multiple imaging techniques are available. Their value, in order of increasing diagnostic importance, is discussed below.

Standard X-Ray Imaging of the Skull and Spinal Column

The main value of standard x-ray imaging of the skull is to detect metallic objects in the facial tissues, eyes, or skull or intracranially before magnetic resonance imaging (MRI). Metal objects, in particular those containing iron, can be moved and become hot during MRI, potentially causing severe damage and even death. Metal objects also can result in severe distortion of MRI signals, making interpretation difficult. While not a routine in my practice, if there is concern about the presence of metals in areas to be imaged with MRI, standard x-rays of those areas should be obtained and MRI either withheld or modified, as indicated.

Computed Tomography (CT) Imaging of the CNS

Severe, major changes of MS can be seen on CT scanning of the brain. Large areas of demyelination may show up as hypointensities. Cerebral atrophy can be detected. In some cases, there may be contrast enhancement of large, active lesions. In general, however, CT imaging of the CNS in MS is of limited value for detecting either disease activity or the extent of lesions.

Magnetic Resonance Imaging

MRI is a generic term that encompasses a variety of different techniques. However, all are based on the ability to induce and detect changes in protons. The most common source of protons is the nuclei of water molecules. Thus, MRI primarily shows changes in the state of water in the CNS. What this means is that lesions seen on MRI are relatively nonspecific, with a long list of diseases, ranging from migraine, to stroke, to infection, to neoplasm, to trauma, to MS, causing "spots." Added to this is the fact that there are changes in water distribution with aging, resulting in the appearance of "lesions." No one should make a diagnosis of MS based only on the presence of "lesions" in the CNS. Unfortunately this is often the case.

Conventional MRI Imaging

MRI techniques can be categorized as conventional and nonconventional based on their use in clinical practice. Conventional MRI imaging has greatly increased our ability not only to diagnose MS but also to follow the course of disease at the tissue level and to determine, to an extent, an individual's response to disease-modifying therapy.[1] However, there often is a disconnect between the degree of change seen on MRI and the clinical picture. This has led to skepticism as to the value of MRI in determining prognosis and evaluating response to treatment. However, lack of an immediate correlation between MRI and clinical findings is to be expected given the incomplete picture of tissue pathology provided by conventional MRI. With evolving nonconventional techniques, described briefly below, greater insight into tissue changes may be provided. What has been shown is that changes on conventional MRI can predict an individual's clinical course.[2,3]

There are great variations in the techniques used to obtain MRI images, making comparisons between MRIs done on different machines and at different institutions difficult. To monitor changes in persons with MS, a standardized, consistent protocol should be used, one that will allow monitoring of lesions over time with minimal variations in technique and head positioning. An excellent MRI protocol for imaging persons with MS is found at the Web site of the Consortium for MS Centers (http://www.mscare.org/cmsc/Vancouver-2003-Guidelines-for-a-standardized-MRI-protocol-for-MS.html). This Web site also contains a recommended report form that should be used by the radiologist to report the findings. Using these recommendations will greatly increase the value of MRIs for you and your patients.

T2, Fast Spin Echo (FSE) and Fluid-Activated Inversion Recovery (FLAIR) Imaging

These techniques show MS lesions as hyperintensities ("white spots"). T2 or FSE also shows spinal fluid as white, making discrimination of MS lesions difficult. However, it is the best technique for detecting lesions in the posterior fossa. Imaging of spinal cord lesions is best done with a technique called T2/STIR imaging, though as the sensitivity of the technique increases, so does the appearance of artifacts. With FLAIR imaging the signals from spinal fluid are blocked or inverted, making spinal fluid appear black. This technique is most valuable in detecting lesions above the tentorium.[4] The pathologic changes underlying T2/FLAIR hyperintensities vary greatly. "Lesions" can represent areas of acute inflammation, demyelination, remyelination, and chronic scarring. Thus, T2/FLAIR lesions represent a history of that person's MS, and a single MRI scan does not allow differentiation of acute from chronic lesions. The appearance of new T2/FLAIR lesions over time, however, would suggest the presence of ongoing CNS inflammation and could, if substantive enough, indicate an insufficient response to disease-modifying therapies (Fig. 4.1).

T1 Imaging

This technique shows lesions of MS as hypointensities, or "black holes." There are two kinds of black holes: ones that are transient and represent areas of edema, which resolve over weeks to months, and permanent ones. The underlying pathologic changes of permanent black holes have

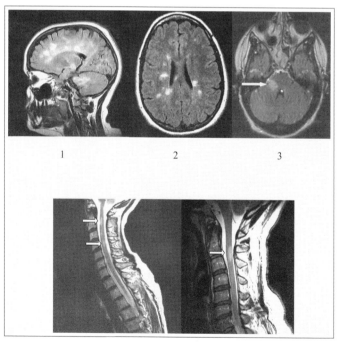

1   2   3

Figure 4.1 Typical T2/FLAIR lesions of MS. Note the periventricular and callosal location of the lesions, their oval shape ("Dawson's fingers"), and the lesions in the right cerebellar peduncle and spinal cord (*arrows*). Images 2 and 3 above and the two images of the spinal cord are courtesy of Tony Traboulsee, MD, University of British Columbia, BC, Canada.

been studied; they have been shown to represent regions of axonal loss.[5,6] The darker the black hole, the more intense the loss of axons (Fig. 4.2). In some individuals with MS most of the lesions noted with T2/FLAIR imaging are hypointense, indicating that their pattern of MS is more tissue destructive. Black hole volume correlates with brain atrophy and with disability better than T2/FLAIR lesion volume and can be an important variable (to be discussed below) in assessing a person's response to treatment.[6] Unfortunately, some radiologists often fail to note such changes in their reports, decreasing the value of their interpretations.

Contrast-Enhancing Lesions

There is a breakdown of the blood–brain barrier in acutely inflamed MS lesions. As a result, substances injected intravenously will "leak" into those areas. If that substance is a magnetically sensitive contrast medium such as gadolinium, it will be detectable on MRI and will appear white. The presence of contrast in an MS lesion indicates that the lesion is less than 8 weeks old.[7] With time lesions lose their contrast enhancement and are visible only on T2/FLAIR or T1 imaging. The pathologic changes of lesions with contrast enhancement are always inflammatory and are usually associated with tissue destruction. In some instances contrast-enhancing lesions are areas of remyelination.

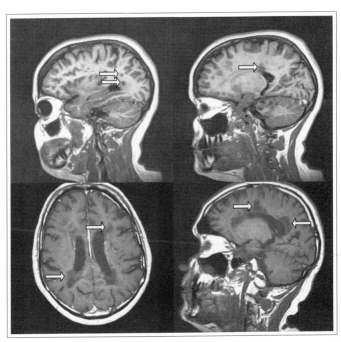

Figure 4.2 Characteristic T1 hypointensities ("black holes"). Arrows point to regions of T1 hypointensity. Note their periventricular and deep cerebral distribution.

Patterns of contrast enhancement vary. Some lesions show a nodular or uniformly dense pattern (left image in Fig. 4.3). Others show a ring of contrast enhancement at the margins ("ring lesions"—right image in Fig. 4.3). Ring-enhancing lesions often are indicative of more intense tissue destruction.

Several caveats must be kept in mind in regard to contrast-enhancing lesions. First, such lesions are transient, so failure to detect contrast enhancement on a single MRI does not indicate disease quiescence. Second, the ability to detect contrast-enhancing lesions varies with the MRI technique. A delay of at least 5 minutes following injection of contrast before reimaging is necessary to allow the contrast to enter the lesions. Imaging done too soon after injection will show many vessels and very few, if any, enhancing lesions. Unfortunately, the incentive of some MRI facilities to image as many patients as possible, in as short a period of time as possible, can result in inadequate assessment of contrast enhancement. Third, the ability to detect contrast enhancement varies with the amount of contrast injected (the higher the dose, the more lesions detected) and with the strength of the MR machine's magnet (expressed as Tesla).[8] The greater the magnet strength, the greater the ability to detect contrast enhancement. Most commercial magnets at this writing have a strength of 1.5 Tesla. However, more machines with 3-Tesla magnets are coming into service, and this may eventually become the standard. Comparing results from 1.5-Tesla and 3-Tesla machines will be difficult at best.

Atrophy

While not a specific MRI technique, CNS atrophy, or loss of tissue substance, can be seen on MRI (Fig. 4.4). Atrophy can be noted in both gray and white matter. CNS atrophy occurs very early in the course of MS, compared to age-matched controls, and correlates well with the degree of disability, both ambulatory ability and cognitive function (see Chapter 3).

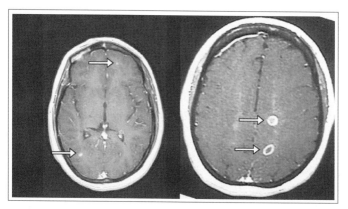

Figure 4.3 Contrast-enhancing lesions of multiple sclerosis. Nodular contrast enhancement (left) and ring contrast enhancement (right). Image at the right is courtesy of Tony Traboulsee, MD.

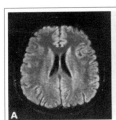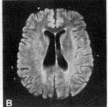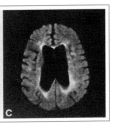

Figure 4.4 Atrophy of the brain in MS. Progressive loss of brain volume over time. Courtesy of Richard Rudick, MD, Cleveland Clinic, Cleveland, OH.

When comparing MRIs visually, changes of greater than 10% in brain or spinal cord volume are necessary to be detected. Thus, assessing CNS atrophy over short periods of time is difficult. Nevertheless, the presence of CNS atrophy is an important indicator of tissue destruction, either from acute inflammation or more indolent inflammation (as described in Chapter 3), and can serve as both a measure of response to disease-modifying therapy and in predicting the clinical course. Techniques for quantifying loss of brain volume automatically are becoming more accessible and may in time become part of the routine clinical evaluation.[9,10] However, decreases in brain volume over the short term may indicate a decrease in CNS inflammation and edema and thus may represent a beneficial effect of a disease-modifying therapy.

Nonconventional MRI Techniques

New techniques are being developed that can provide further insights into the pathogenic tissue changes noted in MS. As of this writing these techniques are not routinely available due to the additional time needed to obtain the data, the complexity of data interpretation, the "research" nature of the techniques, and, perhaps most importantly, the lack of additional reimbursement for performing them. Briefly, the following techniques show the greatest promise:

1. *MR Spectroscopy (MRS):* This technique measures the chemical composition of regions of the white matter and gray matter. By measuring the levels of particular chemicals, information on the integrity of tissue in those regions can be obtained. Most valuable have been studies of n-acetyl aspartate (NAA), a measure of neuronal and axonal health and integrity; choline, a measure of glial integrity; and free lipid compounds, a measure of myelin integrity.[11] MRS has been used to show benefits from administration of disease-modifying therapies, with increases in the concentration of NAA in regions of tissue injury following initiation of treatment.

2. *Diffusion Tensor Imaging (DTI):* This technique measures water movement along fiber tracts. As tracts become damaged and disrupted by the disease process, the diffusion of water along the axes of the tracts changes, and this can be measured. Similar to MRS, DTI could

become a useful means of measuring not only the extent of fiber tract destruction but also the effects of disease-modifying therapies to enhance tract restoration and healing.

3. *Magnetization Transfer Imaging and Magnetic Transfer Ratio (MTR):* This technique measures the ability to transfer energy from protons that are free in solution to protons bound to macromolecules such as myelin and proteins. If tissue integrity is disrupted, transfer of energy is altered. A ratio is obtained of proton energy derived from free water and protons bound to macromolecules: the lower the ratio, the more tissue disruption is present.[5] Using MTR, researchers have shown that even normal-appearing white matter in persons with MS is abnormal compared to white matter in normal individuals. Again, MTR has the potential to show not only the extent of tissue disruption but also the ability of disease-modifying therapies to restore tissue integrity.

4. *Functional MRI (fMRI):* None of the above techniques measures the functional capacity of the brain. fMRI has this ability. It measures changes in the ratios of oxyhemoglobin and deoxygenated hemoglobin in regions of the brain before and after these regions are activated. Oxyhemoglobin concentrations increase in areas of increased blood flow, presumably due to the increased metabolic needs of that region. Thus, the appearance of oxyhemoglobin serves as a surrogate marker for increased neuronal activity. This technique has allowed researchers to show that persons with MS compensate for brain lesions by using other areas of the brain not usually involved in these tasks.[6] This demonstration of brain plasticity may be one reason persons with MS are able to recover after an attack.

5. *Optical Coherence Tomography (OCT):* OCT is not an MRI technique; rather, it is a method of measuring the thickness of the eye's retinal nerve fiber layer using high-resolution analyses of reflected infrared light. The retinal nerve fiber layer consists of nonmyelinated axons derived from neurons in the eye, and changes in this layer could serve as markers for axonal damage in the CNS. There is marked thinning of the retinal nerve fiber layer in eyes affected by optic neuritis. Whether changes in the retinal nerve fiber layer can be used as surrogates for changes to axons in the CNS is the subject of much research. The advantage of OCT is its ease of administration, rapidity, and much lower costs than MRI.

Use of Conventional MRI in the Diagnosis of MS

Localized changes in water content (proton density) can occur with many CNS processes, including such common conditions as migraines, diabetes mellitus, high blood pressure, trauma, infection, neoplasm, and aging. Thus, MS is but one of many diseases that can cause "spots" on MRI. What is critical in corroborating and establishing a diagnosis of MS is not the presence of "spots," but their shape and location.[12]

Since many inflammatory lesions in MS are around veins, MS lesions are often oval and oriented perpendicular to the axes of the ventricles.

When present around ventricles, these lesions have the appearance of fingers, called "Dawson's fingers." An example of such lesions is found in Figure 4.1. In addition to lesion shape, lesion location is of value in supporting a diagnosis of MS. Typically lesions are present adjacent to the lateral ventricles, in the subcortical white matter, in deep white matter, and in both the posterior fossa (brain stem and cerebellum) and the spinal cord. Lesions in the brain stem and spinal cord are uncommon in migraines, high blood pressure, and diabetes mellitus, and the presence of such lesions can support a diagnosis of MS. A case can be made for obtaining spinal cord MRIs in persons suspected of having MS, even in the absence of spinal cord symptoms or signs.

Criteria have been published about the numbers and patterns of T2/FLAIR lesions needed to support a diagnosis of MS (Barkhof criteria[13]— Table 4.1). Since MS is a multifocal CNS disease, more than one lesion must be present and in a characteristic location. For a person presenting with an initial MS-related symptom, changes on MRI establish that the disease process is multifocal, that is "disseminated in space." However, the other criterion that is needed is evidence of disease progression, or "dissemination in time." This must be done to show that the initial illness is not monophasic. The MRI is of value in establishing this, too. According to the newly revised McDonald criteria (see Chapter 5), any new lesion, occurring in a site different from that of the original lesion(s), is considered evidence of disease progression. In most instances a delay of 3 months between MRIs is suggested to allow lesion development. The changes noted are usually new lesions seen on T2/FLAIR imaging, with or without contrast enhancement. Once noted, assuming all other criteria are met, a diagnosis of clinically definite MS is established.

Use of MRI in Predicting the Course of MS

Predicting the course of disease in persons with MS is difficult at best. However, there are data that indicate a role for MRI. Several recent studies have shown that the number of T2/FLAIR lesions in the CNS at onset of disease is a good predictor of clinical course.[2,3] If a person with a clinically isolated syndrome (that is, an individual having a first attack suggestive of a CNS inflammatory process) has only one lesion on MRI, there is still a chance of progressing to clinically definite MS and having an Expanded Disability Status Scale (EDSS) score of 6 more (walking with a cane) after 20 years, but the risk is relatively small (18%). If a person with a clinically

Table 4.1 Barkhof et al.[12] MS MRI Criteria
At least three of the four following changes must be noted:
1. At least one gadolinium-enhancing lesion or nine T2 hyperintense lesions
2. At least one infratentorial (or spinal cord) lesion
3. At least one subcortical lesion
4. At least three periventricular lesions

From Barkhof, Filippi M, Miller DH, et al. Comparison of MRI criteria at first presentation to predict conversion to clinically definite multiple sclerosis. *Brain.* 1997;120(Pt 11):2059–2069.

isolated syndrome presents with more than 10 lesions typical for MS on the initial CNS MRI, there is almost certainty that there will be progression to clinically definite MS in 20 years, with a 60% chance of reaching an EDSS of 6 within that time. Thus, the number of T2/FLAIR lesions noted at disease onset is a predictor of clinical course and can be used as a guide for initiation of treatment.

Use of MRI in Following Response to Disease-Modifying Therapy

This remains a controversial topic among MS experts because of the disconnect between the number of T2/FLAIR lesions seen on MRI and the clinical status of the patient, and the fact that none of the disease-modifying therapies are cures, so new MRI lesions and clinical relapses can occur despite treatment with any of these medications. Using a standardized imaging technique, as noted above, greatly improves the reliability of comparing serial MRIs.

As noted above, not all MRI lesions are equivalent in terms of identifying the extent of tissue destruction.[5] Thus, lesion load per se is not sufficient; more important is the nature of the lesion. The presence or development of new hypointense T1 lesions suggests more intense tissue destruction than would the appearance of new T2/FLAIR lesions that are isointense on T1 imaging. The presence of increasing brain atrophy over relatively short periods of time (1 to 2 years) suggests a poor prognosis. The presence of increasing numbers of lesions with contrast enhancement would indicate a less-than-optimal response to disease-modifying therapy. All of these changes can occur in the absence of clinical changes, indicating sufficient CNS plasticity to allow adaptation. However, plasticity is limited, and eventually there are clinical consequences. Most MS specialists agree that substantive changes in the volume of T2/FLAIR or T1 lesions, increasing brain atrophy, or recurring, increasing numbers of lesions with contrast enhancement would indicate a less-than-optimal response to disease-modifying therapy and a need to reassess that patient for a change in treatment. What remains a source of dispute among MS specialists is the threshold of change needed to determine a less-than-optimal treatment response. There are no absolute criteria, and there may never be, given the variations in disease course, both clinical and on MRI.

Another caveat to using MRI to assess response to disease-modifying therapy is that changes in lesion pattern induced by disease-modifying therapy take time. The MS disease process has "momentum." By that I mean that disease processes occurring at the time of treatment initiation may not be affected by treatment and will continue to evolve, leading to new lesions on MRI or clinical relapses. Thus, an interval of at least 6 to 9 months should be allowed before the efficacy of a treatment is assessed either clinically or on MRI. Even then, there may be continuing and increasing benefit, and switching disease-modifying therapy within a year of initiation should be done only in individuals with clearly relentless disease progression.

As noted previously, the course of MS can change over time, and changes on MRI may predict subsequent clinical changes. This may occur either for unknown reasons or, as will be described in Chapter 8, due to the appearance of neutralizing antibodies to beta-interferon. The question then is, how often one should do MRIs on persons receiving disease-modifying therapy? Again, there are no universally agreed upon standards. My approach is to do MRIs at least annually in persons taking disease-modifying therapy for the first several years, and then, in the presence of disease stability, to do them every several years. Which regions of the CNS are imaged will depend on the person's pattern of disease. In those with both brain and spinal cord lesions, I will image both areas. Brain alone will be imaged in those with previously normal spinal cords.

Since some changes on MRI may occur with any disease-modifying therapies, deciding how much change is necessary to indicate insufficient efficacy remains a matter of clinical judgment. Certainly the appearance of many new T2/FLAIR, T1, or contrast-enhancing lesions in an individual with previously quiescent scans should engender concern.

As relapsing-remitting MS progresses, the acute inflammatory changes that are most visible on MRI become less frequent and less prominent. Thus, the value of MRI in assessing responses to disease-modifying therapy becomes less useful as patients enter the secondary-progressive phase of their illness. Unless continuing clinical relapses are noted or continuing new lesions are seen in persons with a gradually progressive clinical course, I do not do many MRIs on persons in their secondary-progressive phase. Indeed, there are data showing that the T2/FLAIR lesion load decreases over time in persons entering this secondary-progressive phase, possibly as a result of brain atrophy and condensation of lesions around the ventricles.

References

1. Arnold DL. The place of MRI in monitoring the individual MS patient. *J Neurol Sci.* 2007;259:123–127.

2. Brex PA, Ciccarelli O, O'Riordan JI, et al. A longitudinal study of abnormalities on MRI and disability from multiple sclerosis. *N Engl J Med.* 2002;346:158–164.

3. Fisniku LK, Brex PA, Altmann DR, et al. Disability and T2 MRI lesions: a 20-year follow-up of patients with relapse onset of multiple sclerosis. *Brain.* 2008;131:808–817.

4. Bastianello S, Bozzao A, Paolillo, A et al. Fast spin-echo and fast fluid-attenuated inversion-recovery versus conventional spin-echo sequences for MR quantification of multiple sclerosis lesions. *AJNR Am J Neuroradiol.* 1997;18:699–704.

5. van Waesberghe JH, Kamphorst W, De Groot CJ, et al. Axonal loss in multiple sclerosis lesions: magnetic resonance imaging insights into substrates of disability. *Ann Neurol.* 1999;46:747–754.

6. Traboulsee A. MRI relapses have significant pathologic and clinical implications in multiple sclerosis. *J Neurol Sci.* 2007;256(Suppl 1):S19–22.

7. Cotton F, Weiner HL, Jolesz FA, Guttmann CR. MRI contrast uptake in new lesions in relapsing-remitting MS followed at weekly intervals. *Neurology.* 2003;60:640–646.

8. Bachmann R, Reilmann R, Schwindt W, et al. FLAIR imaging for multiple sclerosis: a comparative MR study at 1.5 and 3.0 Tesla. *Eur Radiol.* 2006;16:915–921.

9. De Stefano N, Battaglini M, Smith SM. Measuring brain atrophy in multiple sclerosis. *J Neuroimaging.* 2007;17(Suppl 1):10S–15S.

10. Sharma J, Sanfilipo MP, Benedict RH, et al. Whole-brain atrophy in multiple sclerosis measured by automated versus semiautomated MR imaging segmentation. *AJNR Am J Neuroradiol.* 2004;25:985–996.

11. Ge Y, Gonen O, Inglese M, et al. Neuronal cell injury precedes brain atrophy in multiple sclerosis. *Neurology.* 2004;62:624–627.

12. Barkhof F, Scheltens P. Imaging of white matter lesions. *Cerebrovasc Dis.* 2002;13(Suppl 2):21–30.

13. Barkhof F, Filippi M, Miller DH, et al. Comparison of MRI criteria at first presentation to predict conversion to clinically definite multiple sclerosis. *Brain.* 1997;120(Pt 11):2059–2069.

Further Reading

Amato MP, Portaccio E, Goretti B, et al. Association of neocortical volume changes with cognitive deterioration in relapsing-remitting multiple sclerosis. *Arch Neurol.* 2007;64(8):1157–1161.

Bagnato F, Jeffries N, Richert ND, et al. Evolution of T1 black holes in patients with multiple sclerosis imaged monthly for 4 years. *Brain.* 2003;126(Pt 8):1782–1789.

Bitsch A, Kuhlmann T, Stadelmann C, et al. A longitudinal MRI study of histo-pathologically defined hypointense multiple sclerosis lesions. *Ann Neurol.* 2001;49(6):793–796.

De Stefano N, Cocco E, Lai M, et al. Imaging brain damage in first-degree relatives of sporadic and familial multiple sclerosis. *Ann Neurol.* 2006;59:634–639.

Lebrun C, Bensa C, Debouverie M, et al. Unexpected multiple sclerosis: follow-up of 30 patients with magnetic resonance imaging and clinical conversion profile. *J Neurol Neurosurg Psychiatry.* 2008;79:195–198.

Polman CH, Reingold SC, Edan G, et al. Diagnostic criteria for multiple sclerosis: 2005 revisions to the "McDonald Criteria." *Ann Neurol.* 2005;58:840–846.

Siva A. The spectrum of multiple sclerosis and treatment decisions. *Clin Neurol Neurosurg.* 2006;108:333–338.

Tintore M, Rovira A, Rio J, et al. Baseline MRI predicts future attacks and disability in clinically isolated syndromes. *Neurology.* 2006;67:968–972.

Villar LM, Garcia-Barragan N, Sadaba MC, et al. Accuracy of CSF and MRI criteria for dissemination in space in the diagnosis of multiple sclerosis. *J Neurol Sci.* 2008;266:34–37.

Chapter 5

Making a Diagnosis of Multiple Sclerosis

This chapter will recapitulate, review, and attempt to consolidate the information presented in Chapters 2 through 4 with the intent of allowing the reader to have an algorithm for diagnosing MS.

Despite the advent of sensitive imaging techniques such as MRI and the value of spinal fluid analyses, the diagnosis of MS remains based on clinical criteria. By that I mean there must be symptoms and signs suggestive of multifocal CNS dysfunction. Symptoms alone are insufficient to make the diagnosis, nor is the presence of "typical" changes on MRI or in cerebrospinal fluid sufficient. There should be a confluence of clinical and laboratory data supporting the presence of a chronic, progressive, inflammatory CNS disease, not caused by other more defined infectious, metabolic, vascular, neoplastic, or genetically defined illnesses.

Patterns of Disease Presentation

As discussed in Chapter 3, there are four general patterns of disease progression in MS.[1,2] The most common pattern, noted in about 85% of persons with MS, is one of relapsing and remitting neurologic symptoms. Neurologic symptoms may appear over minutes to hours to days and remit, either partially or completely, over days to months. Intervals between relapses vary greatly, as do degrees of recovery. Next most common is a pattern characterized by the insidious development of neurologic symptoms over weeks to months. Symptoms slowly progress with no true remission but with intermittent periods of disease stability. This pattern is called primary-progressive MS, and the diagnostic criteria for this pattern of disease differ from those of relapsing-remitting MS (see Chapter 3). Primary-progressive MS must be differentiated from secondary-progressive MS, discussed below. Least common, noted at most in only 5% of persons with MS, is a pattern of disease characterized by insidious onset of neurologic difficulties with occasional superimposed relapses and remissions. This pattern is called, appropriately, progressive-relapsing MS. Many persons with relapsing-remitting MS will change their pattern of disease over time to one of gradually progressive neurologic dysfunction with no superimposed relapses. In this pattern individuals note a gradual decrease in relapse frequency (a phase called transitional MS), associated with fewer new and active lesions on MRI. This pattern is called secondary-progressive MS and can occur many years, even decades, following an antecedent relapse. This is important information for the clinician, since recall of one or two minor relapses decades earlier may be difficult and progression of symptoms may be comparable to those noted with primary-progressive MS. However, the pathogenesis and treatment of these two patterns of MS may be different. Thus, every effort should be made to identify any prior acute neurologic episodes in persons with gradually increasing neurologic dysfunction before making a diagnosis of primary-progressive MS.

Demographics

While not essential for making a diagnosis of MS, understanding the demographics of the different patterns of MS is of value. Relapsing-remitting MS is a disease of young adults, usually presenting between the ages of 16 and 50. While individuals outside this age range can develop MS, they are relatively uncommon (see Chapter 11 for a review of pediatric MS). Women predominate at ratios of 2 to 3:1 over men.[3] In the past century there has been a dramatic increase in the incidence of MS, affecting mainly women.[4–7] The reasons for this are not clear but support the hypothesis that changes in the environment are resulting in increased susceptibility to this disease. In contrast to relapsing-remitting MS, primary-progressive MS is most common in adults in their middle years, between ages 40 and 60, with equal ratios of men and women.[8] The demographics of patients with progressive-relapsing MS is similar to those with primary-progressive MS.

Genetics of MS

While the multitude of genes involved in the pathogenesis of MS are not known, they most likely first segregated in Northern Europe. As a result, most persons with MS are either of Northern European origin or have ancestors from that region. As a corollary, while there may be only six degrees of separation between all of us, MS is very rare in certain racial populations. These are well described and include American Indians, African blacks, Hutterites, and Asians. While demyelinating diseases can occur in Asians, their patterns of presentation are different from those of MS, as are their laboratory findings.[9] Further details will be discussed in the section on the differential diagnosis of MS. The genes most associated with susceptibility to MS are those of the major histocompatibility complex, especially the HLA-DR2 genes, but there is sufficient heterogeneity of these genes in persons with MS that they are of no value in terms of diagnosis. Recent human genome-wide studies showed an association of MS with genes of the cytokine receptor IL7R, but this gene accounts for only 2% of disease susceptibility.[10,11] Clearly, multiple genes must be involved in disease susceptibility, disease severity, and pattern of disease.

Initial Clinical Symptoms in Persons with Relapsing-Remitting MS

Individuals presenting with their first episode of CNS dysfunction that has a high probability of evolving into clinically definite MS are said to have a clinically isolated syndrome (CIS). While certain presentations are more common in persons with a CIS, the initial symptoms of relapsing-remitting MS are as varied as the functions of the CNS. None is specific for MS and, as will be repeated throughout this chapter, other illnesses can cause similar symptoms and must be excluded. However, certain symptoms are more common in MS and suggest the possibility of an inflammatory CNS process.

Presenting symptoms often are described both in neurologic terms (numbness, weakness, tremors) and as changes of function, such as increased difficulty with handwriting or doing up buttons, increased difficulty with walking, running, or leg coordination, or difficulty tracking while reading, Such symptoms have diverse possible etiologies, and the diagnostician may need to rely on physical signs for greater clarification. However, in the absence of objective data indicating the presence of CNS dysfunction, one cannot make a diagnosis of MS.[12] In other words, symptoms alone are insufficient to diagnose MS.

Visual Changes

Among the most common presenting symptoms are changes in visual function. These can take the form of monocular (rarely binocular) decreased visual acuity or blurred vision, described as looking through a fogged window or smudged eyeglasses, often involving central vision more than peripheral vision. Less common is a loss of color intensity, with everything appearing "bleached" or lighter. In severe instances vision is lost entirely. If the visual loss results from inflammation of the optic nerve as opposed to a lesion in the optic chiasm, there may be sharp or dull pain behind and over the eye, worse with eye movement, and at times preceding the onset of visual difficulty by days to weeks. In MS, these visual difficulties are most likely the result of an inflammation of the optic nerve (optic neuritis) and can occur over a matter of hours to days, often subsiding completely without treatment over weeks to months. However, degrees of recovery vary.

Sensory Changes

Sensory symptoms as presenting features in MS also are very common. Their onset, in contrast to sensory changes resulting from compressive neuropathies or radiculopathies, is usually painless, with some exceptions. Patterns of sensory change vary widely, at times involving particular dermatomes, such as the C7–T2 dermatomes (medial hands and arms), fingertips, feet, and legs. Sensory symptoms that start in the distal lower extremities, then gradually ascend to the abdomen or chest are common, and often associated with a tightness in the abdomen or thorax ("like a girdle or rope"). Less commonly facial and tongue numbness and tingling are noted. Symptoms may be unilateral or bilateral and can be worsened with fatigue or increased body temperature. The nature of the sensory changes varies, ranging from numbness, to numbness and tingling, to a dysesthetic, uncomfortable, prickling and burning sensation (causalgia). None of these sensory changes is unique to MS, but if they are present bilaterally and are associated with a buzzing, electric, shock-like sensation into the back or limbs upon neck flexion (Lhermitte's sign), this strongly suggests the presence of spinal cord dysfunction. As with visual difficulties, symptoms may spontaneously resolve partially or completely over days to weeks.

Brain Stem Dysfunction

Vertigo and feelings of imbalance or dizziness are some of the most common symptoms in any clinical practice of neurology and can be related to medications, changes in blood pressure, inner ear (vestibular) dysfunction, musculoskeletal abnormalities of the neck ("cervical vertigo"), and of course brain stem dysfunction in MS. The dizziness and vertigo of CNS origin can be positional and worsened with rapid eye movements, but it is unusual for tinnitus and decreased hearing to be part of that symptom complex. Since inflammation of the brain stem in MS often involves other nuclei, the vertigo associated with MS can be associated with other symptoms such as diplopia, oscillopsia, dysarthria, or numbness. Studies of isolated vertigo in persons with MS suggest it is most often due to inner ear dysfunction rather than CNS inflammation, and deciding whether an antecedent episode of vertigo was of central or peripheral origin can be difficult.[13]

Double vision with or without oscillopsia (the symptom of nystagmus, with "bouncing" or jumping vision) can be a presenting symptom in MS. Again, other conditions such as diabetes, vascular disease of the CNS, either ischemic or aneurysmal, myasthenia gravis, and neoplastic processes can cause identical symptoms. In MS the diplopia is usually not associated with any pupillary or eyelid changes and is often present on gaze to either side and vertically. The presence of skew diplopia, or dislocation of objects in the vertical as opposed to horizontal plane, is very suggestive of a CNS origin of the diplopia.

Motor Changes

Weakness is a common presenting symptom in MS. Often symptoms of weakness are noted only in the context of prolonged exertion ("my right leg begins to drag only after I've walked several miles") or with elevations of core body temperature, such as with infections or hot weather. Weakness may involve any part of body but most commonly affects the lower extremities, either proximally or distally. Bilateral lower extremity weakness is most suggestive of spinal cord dysfunction and often is associated with changes in bowel, bladder, or sexual function. There can be changes in tone, with onset of muscle cramping or the appearance of myoclonic jerks, often when lying down at night.

Changes in Energy

One of the most common symptoms of MS is fatigue. It is not the kind of fatigue one has from insufficient rest or sleep that is quickly eased with a nap or a good night's rest. Rather, it is the kind of fatigue one feels after a bout of the flu or other viral infection, namely a more permeating fatigability that is not eased with rest alone and verges on a generalized feeling of weakness. It can vary in degree from mild to severe and can be a major component of disability in MS. A change in energy levels at the time of presentation with any of the above symptoms should make one consider a CNS inflammatory process such as MS as a potential cause. However, fatigue can have multiple causes ranging from hematologic, to metabolic, to endocrine, to psychological, and all these must be considered first (see Chapter 9).

Lower Spinal Cord Dysfunction

Changes in bowel, bladder, and sexual function, occurring in isolation, are unusual in MS, but they frequently occur in association with lower extremity sensory and motor changes, suggesting spinal cord dysfunction. Most common are changes in pattern, with more bladder urgency and frequency, more constipation or alternating constipation and diarrhea, and more difficulty with arousal and orgasm.

Onset of symptoms may be precipitous, occurring over minutes to hours, or insidious, occurring over days, weeks, and months. Most symptoms of MS persist for more than 48 hours, though fluctuations may be considerable, especially when fatigue or elevations of ambient or core temperature are present, as with fever, exercise, or hot baths. Worsening of symptoms with elevations of core temperature (Uthoff's phenomenon) results from an increased conduction block of nerve impulses along already damaged and compromised pathways. Occasionally presenting MS symptoms may be paroxysmal, such as those occurring with trigeminal neuralgia, either unilateral or bilateral, due to an inflammatory nidus in the region of the fifth cranial nerve. Indeed, the onset of bilateral trigeminal neuralgia occurs more frequently in persons with MS.[14,15] Ten percent of persons with MS will have seizures as a result of cortical inflammation, but seizures as a presenting symptom is unusual and should provoke a search for other causes. Even less common are paroxysmal, dystonic, hemicorporal episodes, with sudden flexion of an arm and leg, sparing the face, and often associated with falling. Episodes can last for seconds to minutes and may be provoked by movement. These are believed to be of spinal origin and are usually seen in individuals with antecedent spinal cord dysfunction.[16] It is unusual for a Lhermitte's sign to be a presenting symptom of MS, but it almost always indicates cervical spinal cord dysfunction, either from structural impingement due to cervical spine disease or to intrinsic cervical spinal cord disease. I have seen patients with clinically definite MS who develop a Lhermitte's sign. However, with MRI imaging of the cervical spine, they turned out to have a large cervical disc as a cause of that symptom. In view of the difficulty in distinguishing common neck pain due to musculoskeletal dysfunction, associated with radiating muscle spasms, from the uncomfortable, electrical "buzzing" of Lhermitte's sign precipitated by neck flexion and due to spinal cord dysfunction, an MRI of the cervical spine is necessary.

Initial Clinical Symptoms of Primary-Progressive MS

In contrast to the often precipitous onset of symptoms in persons with relapsing-remitting MS, the onset of symptoms in persons with primary-progressive MS may be so insidious as to preclude determining a time of onset with precision greater than months or years. In addition, visual or cranial nerve symptoms at the onset of primary-progressive MS are unusual, in keeping with the pathophysiology of the disease, which mainly involves the spinal cord.[8] The most common symptoms are those of gradually increasing imbalance, extremity weakness, limb tightness, numbness and tingling of either a limb or limbs, usually the legs, and often the lower trunk, with changes in bowel, bladder, and sexual function, similar to those noted with relapsing-remitting MS. Needless to say, this pattern of neurologic change is not unique to persons with primary progressive MS.

Presenting Signs in Multiple Sclerosis

In general, the findings on the neurologic examination are appropriate to the individual's presenting symptoms. Thus, in persons presenting with the visual difficulties of an optic neuritis, there almost always is decreased visual acuity, not correctable with glasses, with visual field defects, usually in the form of central or paracentral scotomata, loss or decrease of color intensity, especially to red, decreased contrast sensitivity as noted with reading from a Sloan Chart, an afferent papillary defect, and less commonly edema of the optic nerve. Since demyelination of optic nerves can occur subclinically, the presence of optic atrophy or an afferent papillary defect on the neurologic examination, even in the absence of an antecedent history of visual symptoms, can be of great value in identifying the presence of multifocal neurologic dysfunction ("dissemination of neurologic signs in space"). Sensory changes in MS often are not sharply defined as they are with peripheral nervous system abnormalities, except for those associated with transverse spinal cord dysfunction, where sensory levels on the abdomen or thorax can be very sharply demarcated.

The signs in persons presenting with diplopia are most often those of an internuclear ophthalmoplegia (INO) or an abducens weakness. The INO is usually bilateral. The abducens weakness is usually unilateral. Nystagmus is a feature of an INO, yet in my experience it usually is not associated with oscillopsia. Rather, persons describe visual blurring with lateral gaze, trouble with tracking when reading, or a discomfort on lateral gaze that cannot be clearly defined.

Persons with symptoms of limb weakness may have demonstrable weakness on formal testing, with or without associated changes in tone. Muscle tone may be normal or diffusely increased, with or without spasticity. Reflexes are usually increased, and Babinski responses are common.

It is common for the biologic onset of MS to precede the initial clinical presentation.[17] The MRI typically shows much more silent disease than is associated with clinical symptoms and signs, so much so that less than 1 in 10 new T2 or contrast-enhancing lesions is associated with the appearance or worsening of a symptom. As a result, there may be findings on the neurologic examination that were not noted by the individual and were not associated with any symptom. As noted above, this is commonly seen with abnormalities of the optic nerve, where the presence of temporal disc pallor may indicate a subclinical episode of optic neuritis. Equally common are findings of deep tendon reflex asymmetry, usually with disproportionately active reflexes of the lower extremities. At times Babinski responses will be found without associated lower extremity hyperreflexia and increased lower extremity tone. Imbalance or gait ataxia may not be noted by the individual but can be seen when attempting to do tandem gait. The causes of such imbalance are multiple, ranging from poor vision, to sensory loss, to cerebellar dysfunction or weakness, and this finding must be interpreted within these contexts.

Just as the presence of particular symptoms and signs may suggest a diagnosis of MS, their absence can cast the diagnosis in doubt. Rudick et al. suggested a series of "red flag" negatives that should cause a clinician to pause before diagnosing this disease.[18] These include the absence of objective optic nerve or oculomotor findings, the absence of clinical remissions, the absence of sensory findings, the absence of bowel or bladder difficulties, and normal or atypical MRI and cerebrospinal fluid findings. None of these are totally exclusionary, especially early in the course of MS or in persons with variants of MS such as primary-progressive MS. However, in persons with long neurologic histories and many of the above "negatives," a history of diseases other than MS should be considered.

Magnetic Resonance Imaging

The advent of MRI both simplified and complicated the diagnosis if MS (see Chapter 4). MS is a multifocal, progressive, inflammatory disease of the CNS, and MRIs can show these changes. However, the changes seen on MRI are based on changes in proton density ("water content") and thus are intrinsically nonspecific. "Spots" on MRI thus can occur with any condition that results in changes of proton density. These can range from normal aging, to migraine, high blood pressure, head injury, infection, or vasculitis. Thus, changes on MRI should never be used in isolation to make a diagnosis of MS, regardless of what the radiology report may state. That said, there are changes on MRI very suggestive of the diagnosis of MS.

The changes on MRI seen in persons with MS correlate with the gross and histologic pathology of the disease. While lesions of MS can occur anywhere, they are most often periventricular and subcortical. Lesions in the corpus callosum and corona radiata are equally common. Less common are lesions in the posterior fossa, but their presence in this region is atypical for many of the other causes of supratentorial "spots," such as hypertension and migraine, thus reducing the list of possible disease processes. Spinal cord lesions are also common in MS and uncommon in many of the other diseases causing supratentorial changes. Their presence again reduces the list of diagnostic possibilities. Pathologically, changes of MS are common in cortical gray matter and can be very extensive but are poorly, if at all, visible with conventional MRI.

In addition to the location of lesions in MS, their configuration, especially on T2/FLAIR imaging, can be of value. Again, the MRI changes reflect the pathology of the disease. The inflammation of MS is often perivenular, and as a result the lesions of MS may have an elongated or oval appearance. When present in rows along the ventricular edge they are called Dawson's fingers. Many lesions are round, and when present subcortically they have a curved appearance, reflecting the configuration of the subcortical "U fibers." Criteria for the shape and distribution of MRI lesions suggestive of MS are published.[19] As expected, given the relative nonspecificity of the changes seen on MRI, the sensitivity and specificity of such changes for MS is not 100%. Among the more stringent criteria being used are those promulgated by Barkhof et al.[19,20] These are used in the diagnostic algorithm proposed by McDonald et al. and recently modified by Polman et al.,[1] which is discussed below. Table 5.1 lists the Barkhof et al. criteria. While their specificity for MS is high, their sensitivity is of necessity lower, resulting in more false-negative assessments.

The MRI can be configured in multiple ways to give different images of lesions (see Chapter 4). In MS, most lesions are seen with T2/FLAIR imaging. However, other MRI configurations also provide valuable information on the nature of the "spots" seen. With T1 imaging the lesions of MS may appear hypointense, giving rise to so-called black holes. There are two kinds of black holes: those that appear transiently, in areas of acute inflammation, and probably represent focal edema, and those that are permanent. Several studies have shown that permanent black holes represent areas of focal axonal loss.[21–23] The presence of such black holes in the MRI of a person with MS suggests a more destructive pattern of disease, one that can lead to another change on MRI, namely atrophy.

Recent data show that brain atrophy is an early feature of MS. Measures of atrophy are not standardized, and assessing atrophy on MRI can be difficult using only one's eyeballs. However, in some individuals atrophy, in the form of ventricular enlargement, callosal thinning, and sulcal widening, can be seen at the onset of the disease to an extent disproportionate to

Table 5.1 Barkhof Criteria for Aiding in the Diagnosis of MS

At least three of the four following changes must be noted:

1. At least one gadolinium-enhancing lesion or nine T2 hyperintense lesions
2. At least one infratentorial (or spinal cord) lesion
3. At least one subcortical lesion
4. At least three periventricular lesions

From Barkhof, Filippi M, Miller DH, et al. Comparison of MRI criteria at first presentation to predict conversion to clinically definite multiple sclerosis. *Brain.* 1997;120(Pt 11):2059–2069.

the numbers of T2/FLAIR and T1 lesions present. Such observations have led to the hypothesis that the pathophysiology of MS may consist of two linked but separable processes, inflammation and primary degeneration (see Chapter 3).

The acute inflammatory lesions of MS are associated with a breakdown of the blood–brain barrier. Thus, when a compound such as gadolinium is injected into the veins of a person with MS, the material can leak into newly inflamed lesions and be visible on MRI. Enhancement can persist for up to 8 weeks.[24] Such lesions are called contrast enhancing and have been used to assess therapeutic efficacy in multiple clinical trials (see Chapter 8). Contrast-enhancing lesions are not unique to MS and can be seen in any condition associated with a breakdown of the blood–brain barrier. However, the presence of contrast-enhancing lesions in association with multiple T2/FLAIR lesions, in the appropriate distribution and of the appropriate shape, would be supportive of a diagnosis of MS.

There are many caveats to the use of contrast enhancement in both making a diagnosis of MS and establishing the efficacy of treatment. First is the fact that some persons with MS tend to have many contrast-enhancing lesions, while others do not. This pattern of response holds true for extended periods of time. Second, visualization of enhancement is very technique-dependent (e.g., dosage of contrast, scanning time after contrast injection, strength of magnet). Thus, to an extent, the presence or absence of such lesions is an "artifact" of the technique used. It is clear that inflammation and disease progression can occur in the complete absence of contrast enhancement, so the absence of this phenomenon should not exclude a diagnosis of MS.

The MRI is also of great value in predicting which individuals presenting with their first episode of neurologic dysfunction (a clinically isolated syndrome [CIS]) will go on to develop clinically definite MS. Several studies have shown that persons with CIS who have lesions on their brain MRIs compatible with a CNS inflammatory process like MS have a greatly increased risk of developing clinically definite MS, and this risk increases with the number of lesions present: it is almost 100% if more than 10 lesions are present.[25] In addition, the number of lesions seen on MRI at initial presentation is a predictor of the rate of disease progression. Persons with more than 10 lesions on MRI have a greatly increased risk of having a significant disability within 20 years of onset, especially those who continue to accumulate T2/FLAIR lesions.[26]

Evoked Responses

Disease activity in MS occurs subclinically, resulting in physiologic changes in visual, auditory, and sensory pathways without a history of symptoms referable to these pathways. Additionally, both peripheral and central nervous system diseases can cause similar symptoms, and differentiating these two possibilities can be important in making a diagnosis of MS. It is in these contexts that evoked response testing can be useful. Multiple types of evoked responses are possible. The most common are patterned visual evoked responses (PVERs), which measure latencies of nerve conduction in prechiasmatic visual pathways; brain stem auditory evoked responses (BAERs), which measure latencies in brain stem auditory pathways; and somatosensory evoked responses (SSERs), which measure latencies in central somatosensory pathways.

Multiple studies have been done assessing the usefulness of these tests in terms of sensitivity and specificity.[27] The most reliable is the PVER. If retinal abnormalities are excluded, delays in P100 latencies or significant interocular differences in P100 latencies would indicate abnormalities in one or both optic nerves. Changes may also be noted in wave amplitudes and configuration. In isolation, such changes are less specific in terms of defining demyelinating abnormalities of optic nerves. BAERs and SSERs are technically more difficult and more susceptible to artifact, with less specificity for demyelinating processes. In an individual presenting with a CIS and a paucity of findings on the neurologic examination and MRI, finding evidence for subclinical dysfunction of CNS pathways with evoked responses can help in the diagnosis of MS. Similarly, if there is uncertainty as to the anatomic location of visual, auditory, or sensory symptoms, evoked response testing can be of value.

Cerebrospinal Fluid Analysis

In up to 90% of individuals with clinically definite MS, the cerebrospinal fluid (CSF) will show changes of low-grade inflammation. Some changes are measured directly in CSF, such as the IgG concentration and oligoclonal bandings, while others are calculated from measurements of CSF and serum IgG and albumin. Calculated values, using standard formulas, include the IgG index and IgG synthesis rate. The presence of these changes is a function of both the extent of disease and the anatomic location of the inflammatory lesions. Inflammatory foci near ventricular surfaces will result in CSF abnormalities. However, with more extensive involvement of the blood–brain barrier there can be more leakage of blood components into the CSF, with elevations of total protein. When this is present, the specificity of the calculated changes noted above, suggesting the presence of an inflammatory process as occurs in MS, greatly decreases. Early in the course of disease, when CSF changes can be of greatest value in supporting a diagnosis of MS, the CSF can be normal. It then becomes abnormal over time. In up to almost 20% of patients with clinically definite MS the CSF remains normal, perhaps related to differences in the pathogenesis of disease in these individuals. Nevertheless, the presence of a low-grade inflammation in the CSF, in the absence of other diseases (noted below) that could cause similar changes, would support a diagnosis of MS.[28]

The inflammatory changes seen in the CSF of persons with MS are not specific for MS: similar changes can be seen in many other diseases. In addition, these changes must be interpreted in the context that several of the values are calculated rather than measured directly. Their sensitivity and specificity for MS are greatest when blood–brain barrier breakdown is low and total CSF protein is normal. The presence of a significantly elevated total CSF protein, relatively uncommon in MS, gives rise to elevated values of the calculated parameters.[29,30]

The changes most commonly seen in the CSF of persons with MS are shown in Table 5.2.

As noted above, mild elevations in the number of mononuclear cells are fairly common in persons with relapsing-remitting MS and much less common in the less inflammatory stages of MS, such as primary-progressive MS or secondary-progressive MS. Numbers are almost always under 20/mm³, and a level above 50 should prompt a reconsideration of the diagnosis of MS. The majority of cells are lymphocytes or mononuclear cells. In very acute phases of MS, some polymorphonuclear leukocytes can be present.

Increased amounts of IgG in the CSF, in the presence of a normal total protein concentration, are characteristic of any low-grade CNS inflammatory response. Calculated values, based on serum and CSF IgG and total protein, are used to calculate the IgG index and the IgG synthesis rate. Again, with a normal CSF total protein, they suggest the presence of an

Table 5.2 Spinal Fluid Changes in MS

Finding	Description	Usefulness
Mononuclear pleocytosis	<50 cells//mm³ with some PMNs if very acute disease but mostly mononuclear cells	Not very common but useful when present. If >50 cells/mm³, consider a diagnosis other than MS.
Increased IgG concentration	Measures total CSF IgG	Very useful in the presence of a normal total CSF protein
Increased IgG index	A calculated value based on the concentrations of IgG in serum and CSF	Very useful in the presence of a normal total CSF protein
Increased IgG synthesis rate	A calculated value based on the concentrations of IgG in serum and CSF	Very useful in the presence of a normal total CSF protein
Oligoclonal banding	Bands of proteins in the IgG portion of the gel, not seen in serum	Very useful when present but serum must always be used as a comparison. Also, a high incidence of false-negative results if proper assay techniques, namely isoelectric focusing and immunofixation, are not used.
Myelin basic protein (MBP) elevations	Increased concentrations of an important structural myelin protein	Not very useful since results usually are normal. Will be elevated in cases with more acute, widespread disease. Also not specific for inflammatory states since any destructive myelin process will result in MBP elevations.

in situ inflammatory response in the CNS. The increased concentrations of IgG in the CSF of persons with MS result from increases in particular subpopulations of IgG rather than a general increase in all antibodies. When tested in an appropriate fashion, the presence of these increased subpopulations of antibodies is shown by the presence of oligoclonal bands, which are present in CSF but not in serum. Proper technique is essential to maximize the sensitivity of detecting such bands. The assay should involve isoelectric focusing of the proteins followed by immunofixation.[29,30]

Ruling Out "MS Look-alikes"

As noted initially, none of the historical, physical, or laboratory changes of MS is unique to the disease, so every effort must be made to exclude diseases that can mimic MS. Most can be excluded by simple blood or CSF tests. Others, especially those involving genetic mutations, require more sophisticated and expensive testing. In addition, there are demyelinating diseases that have a different clinical course than MS and probably have a different pathogenesis.

Acute Disseminated Encephalomyelitis

The most common of the non-MS demyelinating diseases is acute disseminated encephalomyelitis (ADEM). While usually a disease of children, occurring after a viral infection, the disease can occur in adults and is associated with multifocal neurologic signs and symptoms, very similar to those noted above in persons with MS.[31] In addition, the MRIs of persons with ADEM can resemble those of persons with MS, though usually the changes are more extensive (Fig. 5.1). However, in addition to the neurologic findings, persons with ADEM can have systemic signs of inflammation, with

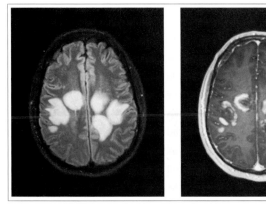

Figure 5.1 MRIs from an adult with ADEM. (*Left*) T2/FLAIR imaging of the extensive, "puffy" lesions widely distributed. (*Right*) Prominent "ring" contrast enhancement of the lesions noted in A. While this pattern can be seen in persons with very acute MS, such findings, in the proper clinical setting, are supportive of a diagnosis of ADEM.

fever, altered levels of consciousness, and leukocytosis. The CSF in ADEM often is more intensely inflammatory than in MS. Most importantly, ADEM is a monophasic illness. Once the disease has run its course—and this may take several months—there should be no new physical signs and the MRI should remain stable.

Differentiating acute MS from ADEM can be difficult, and follow-up over time may be the only way to separate the two illnesses. Recurrences noted after 3 months of onset are most likely due to MS.

Neuromyelitis Optica or Devic's Disease

As the name suggests, neuromyelitis optica (NMO) is a demyelinating/necrotizing disease of the optic nerves and the spinal cord[32,33] (see Chapter 3). The pattern of disease is very variable, with either optic nerve or spinal cord presentations predominating, and with different temporal patterns. Some persons present with recurrent bouts of transverse myelopathy of varying severity. Others have predominantly visual difficulties, either unilateral or bilateral. Degrees of recovery vary widely, but with the more acute, necrotizing form of the disease, severe neurologic deficits can persist.

The pathology of NMO differs from that of MS. Cerebral signs and symptoms are absent and the brain MRI can be normal. The characteristic MRI changes of NMO in the spinal cord are long, contiguous T2/STIR lesions involving multiple cord segments (see Fig. 5.2). The CSF often is more inflammatory than that seen in MS in terms of the number of white blood cells (more than 50/mm^3) and with breakdown of the blood–brain barrier, often without oligoclonal bands. Pathologically, there is an inflammatory vasculitis, associated with the presence of B cells, antibodies, and complement. Recently, an antibody (NMO-IgG) to a ubiquitous water channel protein, aquaporin 4, has been described that is both sensitive and

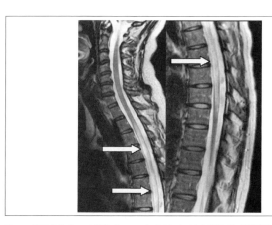

Figure 5.2 Spinal cord MRIs from an individual with NMO. On T2/STIR imaging, contiguous, elongated regions of hyperintensity are noted spanning multiple spinal cord segments. Multiple T2/STIR lesions can be seen in the spinal cords of persons with MS, but rarely do they span multiple segments. MRIs courtesy of Tony Traboulsee, MD, University of British Columbia, BC, Canada.

relatively specific for NMO.[34] While not present in all cases, the presence of NMO-IgG would support this diagnosis.

Other uncommon demyelinating disease include Balo's concentric sclerosis and Marburg's disease, but these are probably variations of MS, differentiated mainly on the basis of the MRI findings (MRIs in persons with Balo's concentric sclerosis show concentric circles of T2 lesions) and the acuteness of the clinical course (very acute in Marburg's disease). No data at this time allow one to separate these illnesses on the basis of differences in pathophysiology.

Other "MS Look-alikes"

A partial list of infectious, inflammatory, genetic, and neoplastic diseases that can mimic MS and that should be considered before making a diagnosis of MS is presented in Table 5.3. This list is by no means inclusive, since more than 100 look-alikes are described. Rather, it lists the most common look-alikes, though none is truly common. Indeed, in the case of Lyme disease, one series from a geographic area where this disease is endemic failed

Table 5.3 Some MS Look-Alikes

Disease	Description	Diagnostic Testing Required
Lyme disease	CNS involvement is seen in the tertiary form of this disease, with multifocal CNS and peripheral nervous system findings and inflammatory changes on MRI and in CSF.	Testing for the presence of antibodies in CSF and serum. Since false-positives can occur in response to other spirochetes, if antibodies are present, Western blots should be obtained to look for patterns of antibody banding specific for infection with *Borrelia bergdorferi*. PCR testing of the CSF for the presence of *Borrelia* antigens can also be of value.
Sjögren's syndrome	A systemic autoimmune disease with ocular, buccal, and joint abnormalities	Dry eyes and mouth are prominent, as are swallowing difficulties. Diagnosis is made with salivary gland or lip biopsy or testing for SSA and SSB antibodies.
Sarcoid	A systemic inflammatory disease of the lungs, skin, joints, and other organs	Causes an inflammatory meningitis, often basilar, affecting cranial nerves and spinal cord. MRIs show meningeal involvement. Diagnosis is made with biopsy of affected non-CNS organs and by the presence of elevated levels of angiotensin-converting enzyme (ACE) in blood and CSF.
Primary CNS vasculitis	An autoimmune vasculitis affecting only the CNS	Can cause relapsing, multifocal CNS signs and symptoms, often stroke-like in nature, affecting both gray and white matter. Can be diagnosed with cerebral angiography, meningeal biopsy, and the presence of various autoantibodies.

Table 5.3 *continued*		
CNS syphilis	Caused by chronic CNS infection with *Treponema pallidum*	Can cause optic nerve and spinal cord injury, usually chronically progressive but with the vascular form of infection more rapid in onset. Diagnosed by the presence of serum and CSF FTA-antibodies.
B12 deficiency	Caused by a deficiency of B12 absorption or a deficiency of a cyanocobalamin carrier protein	Can cause both optic nerve and spinal cord dysfunction. Usually a subacute disease with normal MRI and a non-inflammatory CSF with low B12 levels.
Cerebral autosomal dominant arteriopathy with subcortical infarcts and leukoencephalopathy (CADASIL)	Results from an autosomal dominant mutation in the Notch 3 gene, causing a microangiopathy with associated migraines and often cognitive impairment. Involves both gray and white matter.	MRIs can look very similar to MS but CSF is usually noninflammatory and headaches are a prominent feature of the illness. Can cause a "stuttering," stroke-like progression of symptoms, with evidence of basal ganglia dysfunction too. Diagnosed with genetic testing for Notch 3 gene mutations and family history.
CNS lymphoma	Multifocal infiltrating tumor of the brain can cause progressive multifocal neurologic difficulties, responsive to steroids.	Usually older individuals without a relapsing-remitting course; CSF is noninflammatory but has malignant cells. Brain biopsy may be needed at times.

to show infection with *Borrelia bergdorferi* in any patient originally thought to have MS. In addition, the concept of "chronic" CNS Lyme disease has been called into serious question,[35] negating the need for long-term antibiotic therapies in persons with MS, as advocated by proponents of this concept.

Having MS does not, of course, exclude the possibility of having another illness too, and this must always be considered in the differential diagnosis. For example, a person with MS may have, in addition to MS-related spinal cord dysfunction, a compressive myelopathy due to a disc or neoplasm. Similarly, in persons with MS on immune suppressant medications for illnesses such as organ transplants, or those with immune deficiency diseases such as infection with HIV, superinfections, either viral or bacterial, can mimic acute or subacute "relapses" of disease. Additional studies such as repeat MRI scans, CSF analyses, and even brain biopsy may be needed for differentiation. This may be especially important if progressive multifocal leukoencephalopathy (PML) is suspected. This complication of HIV infection and some disease modifying therapies can result in MRI changes very similar to those of MS.

While not truly an MS look-alike, migraines can cause MRI changes very similar to those seen in MS. Since migraine is a common illness of young adults, many persons with MS also will have this disorder. Discerning which lesions on MRI are due to MS and which may be due to migraines can be a challenge. The presence of contrast enhancement and of T1 hypointensities would favor the cause being MS.

Another illness often confounding the diagnosis of MS is diabetes mellitus, both juvenile and adult onset. Neuropathic, myopathic, and autonomic symptoms can be very similar to those of MS, with sensory changes, weakness, and bowel and bladder dysfunction.[36] Evidence of inflammatory changes on MRI, with contrast enhancement, and in CSF, with the presence of oligoclonal bands, are uncommon in diabetes. Spinal fluid total proteins are commonly elevated in persons with diabetes mellitus. Thus, as noted previously, calculated values of the IgG synthesis rate or the IgG index are much less specific for the presence of CNS inflammation in such a setting.

In our MS specialty clinic up to 25% of individuals presenting with a plethora of symptoms suggestive of multifocal CNS dysfunction do not have MS or another discernible CNS pathologic process. They have normal or functional neurologic examinations, normal CNS MRIs, normal blood tests, and normal CSF. Such individuals are usually categorized as having a somatization disorder, hypochondriasis, or conversion reaction; many such individuals are also clinically depressed. Despite the complexity and severity of their symptoms and associated disabilities, a diagnosis of MS on symptoms alone should not be made.

Early, accurate diagnosis of MS is important so that diseases that may be amenable to other treatments can be excluded and also so that treatment with immune-modulating therapies can be started as early as possible. As described in Chapter 2, MS is a complex illness with different pathogenic processes probably occurring concomitantly. Since the inflammatory component of MS predominates early in the course of the disease in most individuals with relapsing-remitting MS, treatment with anti-inflammatory, immune-modulating therapy is most effective early in the course of the disease .

Algorithms for the Diagnosis of MS

Several algorithms have been published to assist in establishing the diagnosis of MS. Their intent is to provide uniformity to the diagnosis of a disease as pleomorphic as MS and to allow the diagnosis to be made with accuracy as early in the course of disease as possible. This is especially true for individuals who present with their first episode of neurologic dysfunction (that is, those with a CIS). Many such individuals will progress to clinically definite MS, so identifying them early, and if appropriate starting immune-modulating therapy, is important.

The most commonly used algorithms are those published by Poser et al.[37] (Table 5.4) and McDonald et al.,[1] the latter recently revised (Table 5.5). The former uses clinical, laboratory, and imaging criteria to establish the presence of an inflammatory disease of the CNS that is disseminated in time and space. The latter uses the same clinical, laboratory, and imaging criteria but takes into account imaging data subsequent to the first

Table 5.4 Summary of the Poser Committee's Criteria for the Diagnosis of MS

Diagnosis	Clinical Episodes	Neurologic Exam	Imaging Data	CSF Analyses
Clinically definite MS	2	2 anatomic sites of neurologic dysfunction		
	2	1 anatomic site of neurologic dysfunction	≥1 separate lesions not explaining the site of neurologic dysfunction	
Laboratory-supported definite MS	2	1 anatomic site of neurologic dysfunction *or* ≥1 separate lesion not explaining the site of neurologic dysfunction		Immunologic abnormalities compatible with MS
	1	2 anatomic sites of neurologic dysfunction		Immunologic abnormalities compatible with MS
	1	1 anatomic site of neurologic dysfunction *or* ≥1 separate lesion not explaining the site of neurologic dysfunction		Immunologic abnormalities compatible with MS
Clinically probable MS	2	1 anatomic site of neurologic dysfunction		
	1	2 anatomic sites of neurologic dysfunction		
	1	1 anatomic site of neurologic dysfunction *or* ≥1 separate lesion not explaining the site of neurologic dysfunction		
Laboratory-supported probable MS	2			Immunologic abnormalities compatible with MS

neurologic episode to establish dissemination of disease in time and space. Both sets of criteria make it essential to first exclude other possible causes of neurologic illness. The Poser criteria categorize diagnostic certainty into four groups, listed below. The McDonald criteria use three categories of diagnosis: definite MS, possible MS, and not MS. Details of each of the algorithms can be obtained from the articles.

As expected, the correlation between two sets of criteria is not 100% in terms of establishing the diagnosis of clinically definite MS. Several recent prospective studies addressed this question and compared the sensitivity of the two criteria in CIS patients followed for up to 3 years. In one study, which looked at individuals with a CIS, the rate of conversion from CIS to clinically definite MS was 2.4 times higher at the end of 1 year using

Table 5.5 Summary of the Revised McDonald Committee's Criteria for the Diagnosis of MS

	Clinical Settings/Conditions	Attacks	Lesions Suggestive of MS (see above criteria)	Criteria Proven	Additional Clinical or Laboratory Evidence Required if Clinical Evidence Is Insufficient Dissem. in Space	Dissem. in Time
1	Definite MS on clinical grounds	≥2	≥2	Dissem. in time and space	Proven	Proven
2	Localized disease	≥2	1	Dissem. in time	Three of the following: 1. At least one gadolinium-enhancing lesion or nine T2 hyperintense lesions if there is no gadolinium-enhancing lesion. Enhancement of spinal cord lesions also counts. 2. At least one infratentorial lesion, with spinal cord lesions counting in this regard 3. At least one juxtacortical lesion 4. At least three periventricular lesions and 5. (+) CSF	Proven
3	Multifocal attack (can be initial presenting attack or CIS too)	1	≥2	Dissem. in space	Proven	New T2 or enhancing lesion suggestive of MS or a second attack

Table 5.5 (Continued)

Clinical Evidence at Presentation			Additional Clinical or Laboratory Evidence Required if Clinical Evidence Is Insufficient
4	First, monosymptomatic episode (CIS)	1	Three of the following: 1. At least one gadolinium-enhancing lesion or nine T2 hyperintense lesions if there is no gadolinium-enhancing lesion. Enhancement of spinal cord lesions also counts. 2. At least one infratentorial lesion, with spinal cord lesions counting in this regard 3. At least one juxtacortical lesion 4. At least three periventricular lesions and 5. (+) CSF
		1	
		Neither	New T2 or enhancing lesion suggestive of MS or a second attack
5	Primary-progressive MS	Insidious onset with gradual progression of neurologic deficits	Multiple T2 lesions with or without (+) CSF and abnormal PVERs
			New T2 or enhancing lesion suggestive of MS, at least 3 months later, or clinical progression for ≥1 year

the McDonald criteria compared to the Poser criteria, indicating that subclinical changes on MRI were more sensitive than clinical changes in detecting disease progression.[38–40] Thus, the McDonald guidelines could allow the earlier institution of disease-modifying therapy. However, in the study by Dalton et al.,[38] after 3 years of follow-up there were still 28% of patients diagnosed with clinically definite MS by the McDonald criteria who had not met the Poser criteria. These individuals could still develop additional clinical episodes at a later date, thus fulfilling the Poser criteria, but their rate of clinical as opposed to MRI progression was not known. An important caveat of this study was that CSF findings were not used in either of the diagnostic algorithms.

In the study by Fangerau et al.,[39] clinically definite MS was diagnosed more often using the McDonald criteria compared to the "clinically definite" criteria defined by Poser et al. However, when both "clinically definite" and "laboratory-supported definite" criteria were used, the Poser guidelines yielded a higher percentage of definite MS.

In summary, using both clinical and laboratory assessments, the McDonald criteria allow the diagnosis of clinically definite MS to be made earlier, thus allowing the earlier initiation of disease-modifying drugs and ideally having a more salubrious effect on the disease.

Imparting a Diagnosis of MS

Imparting a diagnosis of MS to an individual or family can be either a traumatic or a relieving experience and will vary greatly depending on how the diagnosis is delivered and the background of the patient and the physician. In my years of running an MS specialty clinic I have heard many tales of both "botched" diagnosis and insensitive, even professionally inappropriate, ways of telling individuals they have MS. An example was the patient who was told over the telephone that the MRI showed changes of MS, that there was no cure or effective treatment for this illness, and that the patient should seek care elsewhere. Given the amount of misinformation about MS present in the general population, and the almost inevitable association of "MS" with "wheelchair," every effort should be made to talk with the individual face to face and to provide accurate, complete, compassionate, and most importantly hopeful and encouraging information about the illness.

That said, there are at least three general categories of reactions when patients are told they do or do not have multiple sclerosis. The most common is in persons in whom the diagnosis was not suspected and who, upon hearing it, "glaze over" with fear and sadness, and do not listen to much else that is explained thereafter. Information can be given about Web sites of major, MS patient-oriented, nonprofit organizations, as well as a cautionary word about the amount of misinformation posted on the Internet. In my practice, patients are urged to call with any questions, and I always arrange follow-up appointments within 2 to 3 months to review the course of their illness, discuss treatment options, or evaluate their responses to treatment.

Follow-up MRIs of brain and spinal cord are also scheduled when appropriate to monitor subclinical disease and response to treatment.

The second category of response in persons diagnosed with MS is one of relief. These are individuals with a multitude of difficulties that were never correctly identified and who were either told "there's nothing wrong with you" or were afraid they might have even more potentially disabling illnesses such as a malignant brain tumor or amyotrophic lateral sclerosis. Providing support and information to such individuals is the same in our practice as the first group.

The last pattern of response is one that occurs in persons told they do not have MS. As noted above, about 25% of persons referred to my MS clinic for a second opinion regarding a diagnosis of MS do not meet the diagnostic criteria. These are usually persons with a multitude of somatic complaints, with or without "spots" on MRI, and normal neurologic examinations. They come seeking a diagnosis of definable organic disease to explain their symptoms and can be as disappointed and angry about not having MS as are patients with this illness. I make every effort to reassure persons without MS that not every illness can be neatly defined and that there is more harm in putting someone into the wrong "diagnostic cubbyhole" than in just admitting you cannot explain their difficulties. Symptomatic management of such patients can be very successful, with referral or additional diagnostic testing only when diseases such as cerebral autosomal dominant arteriopathy with subcortical infarcts and leukoencephalopathy (CADASIL) or other MS-mimicking diseases need to be excluded.

References

1. Polman CH, Reingold SC, Edan G, et al. Diagnostic criteria for multiple sclerosis: 2005 revisions to the "McDonald Criteria." *Ann Neurol.* 2005;58:840–846.

2. Lublin FD, Reingold SC. Defining the clinical course of multiple sclerosis: results of an international survey. National Multiple Sclerosis Society (USA) Advisory Committee on Clinical Trials of New Agents in Multiple Sclerosis. *Neurology.* 1996;46:907–911.

3. Orton SM, Herrera BM, Yee IM, et al. Sex ratio of multiple sclerosis in Canada: a longitudinal study. *Lancet Neurol.* 2006;5:932–936.

4. Alonso A, Jick SS, Olek MJ, Hernan MA. Incidence of multiple sclerosis in the United Kingdom: findings from a population-based cohort. *J Neurol.* 2007;254:1736–1741.

5. Debouverie M, Pittion-Vouyovitch S, Louis S, et al. Increasing incidence of multiple sclerosis among women in Lorraine, Eastern France. *Mult Scler.* 2007;13:962–967.

6. Grimaldi LM, Palmeri B, Salemi G, et al. High prevalence and fast-rising incidence of multiple sclerosis in Caltanissetta, Sicily, southern Italy. *Neuroepidemiology.* 2007;28:28–32.

7. Pugliatti M, Riise T, Sotgiu MA, et al. Increasing incidence of multiple sclerosis in the province of Sassari, northern Sardinia. *Neuroepidemiology.* 2005;25:129–134.

8. Miller DH, Leary SM. Primary-progressive multiple sclerosis. *Lancet Neurol.* 2007;6:903–912.

9. Kira J. Multiple sclerosis in the Japanese population. *Lancet Neurol.* 2003;2:117–127.

10. Gregory SG, Schmidt S, Seth P, et al. Interleukin 7 receptor alpha chain (IL7R) shows allelic and functional association with multiple sclerosis. *Nat Genet.* 2007;39:1083–1091.

11. Hafler DA, Compston A, Sawcer S, et al. Risk alleles for multiple sclerosis identified by a genomewide study. *N Engl J Med.* 2007;357:851–862.

12. Levy DE. Transient CNS deficits: a common, benign syndrome in young adults. *Neurology.* 1988;38:831–836.

13. Frohman EM, Kramer PD, Dewey RB, et al. Benign paroxysmal positioning vertigo in multiple sclerosis: diagnosis, pathophysiology and therapeutic techniques. *Mult Scler.* 2003;9:250–255.

14. Hooge JP, Redekop WK. Trigeminal neuralgia in multiple sclerosis. *Neurology.* 1995;45:1294–1296.

15. Jensen TS, Rasmussen P, Reske-Nielsen E. Association of trigeminal neuralgia with multiple sclerosis: clinical and pathological features. *Acta Neurol Scand.* 1982;65:182–189.

16. Ostermann PO, Westerberg CE. Paroxysmal attacks in multiple sclerosis. *Brain.* 1975;98:189–202.

17. Lebrun C, Bensa C, Debouverie M, et al. Unexpected multiple sclerosis: follow-up of 30 patients with magnetic resonance imaging and clinical conversion profile. *J Neurol Neurosurg Psychiatry.* 2008;79:195–198.

18. Rudick RA, Schiffer RB, Schwetz KM, Herndon RM. Multiple sclerosis. The problem of incorrect diagnosis. *Arch Neurol.* 1986;43:578–583.

19. Barkhof F, Filippi M, Miller DH, et al. Comparison of MRI criteria at first presentation to predict conversion to clinically definite multiple sclerosis. *Brain.* 1997;120(Pt 11):2059–2069.

20. Barkhof F, Scheltens P. Imaging of white matter lesions. *Cerebrovasc Dis.* 2002;13(Suppl 2):21–30.

21. Bagnato F, Jeffries N, Richert ND, et al. Evolution of T1 black holes in patients with multiple sclerosis imaged monthly for 4 years. *Brain.* 2003;126:1782–1789.

22. Traboulsee A. MRI relapses have significant pathologic and clinical implications in multiple sclerosis. *J Neurol Sci.* 2007;256(Suppl 1):S19–22.

23. van Waesberghe JH, Kamphorst W, De Groot CJ, et al. Axonal loss in multiple sclerosis lesions: magnetic resonance imaging insights into substrates of disability. *Ann Neurol.* 1999;46:747–754.

24. Cotton F, Weiner HL, Jolesz FA, Guttmann CR. MRI contrast uptake in new lesions in relapsing-remitting MS followed at weekly intervals. *Neurology.* 2003;60:640–646.

25. Brex PA, Ciccarelli O, O'Riordan JI, et al. A longitudinal study of abnormalities on MRI and disability from multiple sclerosis. *N Engl J Med.* 2002;346:158–164.

26. Fisniku LK, Brex PA, Altmann DR, et al. Disability and T2 MRI lesions: a 20-year follow-up of patients with relapse onset of multiple sclerosis. *Brain.* 2008;131:808–817.

27. Sanders EA, Reulen JP, Hogenhuis LA, van der Velde EA. Electrophysiological disorders in multiple sclerosis and optic neuritis. *Can J Neurol Sci.* 1985;12:308–313.

28. Sastre-Garriga J, Tintore M, Rovira A, et al. Conversion to multiple sclerosis after a clinically isolated syndrome of the brainstem: cranial magnetic

resonance imaging, cerebrospinal fluid and neurophysiological findings. *Mult Scler.* 2003;9:39–43.

29. Blennow K, Fredman P, Wallin A, et al. Formulas for the quantitation of intra-thecal IgG production. Their validity in the presence of blood-brain barrier damage and their utility in multiple sclerosis. *J Neurol Sci.* 1994;121:90–96.

30. Luque FA, Jaffe SL. Cerebrospinal fluid analysis in multiple sclerosis. *Int Rev Neurobiol.* 2007;79:341–356.

31. Tenembaum S, Chitnis T, Ness J, Hahn JS. Acute disseminated encephalomyelitis. *Neurology.* 2007;68:S23–36.

32. Argyriou AA, Makris N. Neuromyelitis optica: a distinct demyelinating disease of the central nervous system. *Acta Neurol Scand.* 2008 March 11 [E-pub before print].

33. Wingerchuk DM, Weinshenker BG. Neuromyelitis optica. *Curr Treat Options Neurol.* 2008;10:55–66.

34. Weinshenker BG, Wingerchuk DM. Neuromyelitis optica: clinical syndrome and the NMO-IgG autoantibody marker. *Curr Top Microbiol Immunol.* 2008;318:343–356.

35. Feder HM, Jr., Johnson BJ, O'Connell S, et al. A critical appraisal of "chronic Lyme disease." *N Engl J Med.* 2007;357:1422–1430.

36. Manschot SM, Biessels GJ, Rutten GE, et al. Peripheral and central neurologic complications in type 2 diabetes mellitus: no association in individual patients. *J Neurol Sci.* 2008;264:157–162.

37. Poser CM, Paty DW, Scheinberg L, et al. New diagnostic criteria for multiple sclerosis: guidelines for research protocols. *Ann Neurol.* 1983;13:227–231.

38. Dalton CM, Brex PA, Miszkiel KA et al. Application of the new McDonald criteria to patients with clinically isolated syndromes suggestive of multiple sclerosis. *Ann Neurol.* 2002;52:47–53.

39. Fangerau T, Schimrigk S, Haupts M, et al. Diagnosis of multiple sclerosis: comparison of the Poser criteria and the new McDonald criteria. *Acta Neurol Scand.* 2004;109:385–389.

40. Tintore M, Rovira A, Rio J, et al. New diagnostic criteria for multiple sclerosis: application in first demyelinating episode. *Neurology.* 2003;60:27–30.

Further Reading

Bitsch A, Kuhlmann T, Stadelmann C, et al. A longitudinal MRI study of histopathologically defined hypointense multiple sclerosis lesions. *Ann Neurol.* 2001;49(6):793–796.

Brex PA, Jenkins R, Fox NC, et al. Detection of ventricular enlargement in patients at the earliest clinical stage of MS. *Neurology.* 2000;54(8):1689–1691.

Bruck W, Lucchinetti C, Lassmann H. The pathology of primary progressive multiple sclerosis. *Mult Scler.* 2002;8(2):93–97.

Coyle PK. *Borrelia burgdorferi* antibodies in multiple sclerosis patients. *Neurology.* 1989;39(6):760–761.

Coyle PK, Krupp LB, Doscher C. Significance of reactive Lyme serology in multiple sclerosis. *Ann Neurol.* 1993;34(5):745–747.

De Stefano N, Cocco E, Lai M, et al. Imaging brain damage in first-degree relatives of sporadic and familial multiple sclerosis. *Ann Neurol.* 2006;59(4):634–639.

Ge Y, Gonen O, Inglese M, et al. Neuronal cell injury precedes brain atrophy in multiple sclerosis. *Neurology*. 2004;62(4):624–627.

Johnson MD, Lavin P, Whetsell WO Jr. Fulminant monophasic multiple sclerosis, Marburg's type. *J Neurol Neurosurg Psychiatry*. 1990;53(10):918–921.

Lucchinetti C, Bruck W. The pathology of primary progressive multiple sclerosis. *Mult Scler*. 2004;10(Suppl 1):S23–30.

Lucchinetti CF, Bruck W, Lassmann H. Evidence for pathogenic heterogeneity in multiple sclerosis. *Ann Neurol*. 2004;56(2):308.

Lycklama G, Thompson A, Filippi M, et al. Spinal-cord MRI in multiple sclerosis. *Lancet Neurol*. 2003;2(9):555–562.

Miller D, Barkhof F, Frank JA, et al. Clinically isolated syndromes suggestive of multiple sclerosis, part I: natural history, pathogenesis, diagnosis, and prognosis. *Lancet Neurol*. 2005;4(5):281–288.

Miller D, Barkhof F, Montalban X, et al. Clinically isolated syndromes suggestive of multiple sclerosis, part 2: non-conventional MRI, recovery processes, and management. *Lancet Neurol*. 2005;4(6):341–348.

Miller DH, Barkhof F, Montalban X, et al. Measurement of atrophy in multiple sclerosis: pathological basis, methodological aspects and clinical relevance. *Brain*. 2002;125(Pt 8):1676–1695.

Morioka C, Komatsu Y, Tsujio T, et al. The evolution of the concentric lesions of atypical multiple sclerosis on MRI. *Radiat Med*. 1994;12(3):129–133.

Poser CM. The dissemination of multiple sclerosis: a Viking saga? A historical essay. *Ann Neurol*. 1994;36(Suppl 2):S231–243.

Pulicken M, Gordon-Lipkin E, Balcer LJ, et al. Optical coherence tomography and disease subtype in multiple sclerosis. *Neurology*. 2007;69(22):2085–2092.

Ramirez-Lassepas M, Tulloch JW, Quinones MR, et al. Acute radicular pain as a presenting symptom in multiple sclerosis. *Arch Neurol*. 1992;49(3):255–258.

Strony LP, Wagner K, Keshgegian AA. Demonstration of cerebrospinal fluid oligoclonal banding in neurologic diseases by agarose gel electrophoresis and immunofixation. *Clin Chim Acta*. 1982;122(2):203–212.

Chapter 6

Complications and Comorbidities of Multiple Sclerosis

MS is primarily a disease of the CNS, but as a result of the disease process other organs are often affected. Such changes are often the result of increasing disability and the consequences of this disability. The most important complications and comorbidities are noted below.

Loss of Bone Density (Osteopenia or Osteoporosis)

Loss of bone density is a common complication of persons with MS. It correlates with a loss in the ability to ambulate and bear weight, but occurs to a greater extent even in individuals still able to walk.[1–4] With decreased ability to walk comes a greatly increased risk of falling, and as bone mineral density decreases, so does the risk of fractures. Such fractures often heal poorly and contribute to further disability and increased morbidity and mortality, often requiring expensive surgical procedures and hospitalizations.

In addition to the risks of a decreased ability to bear weight, many MS patients require either multiple short-term or long-term courses of corticosteroids. These drugs can also decrease bone mineral density. Additional factors contributing to decreased bone mineral density are age, smoking, poor diet, lack of exposure to sunlight as individuals become more housebound, lower levels of vitamin D, and loss of estrogens as women enter menopause.

Bone density loss can occur quickly, so early detection is of importance. This is especially the case as persons reach a disability level of being unable to independently walk for 100 feet, and as they begin to require assistive devices (canes, walkers, or braces).

The most useful technique to detect decreased bone mineral density is double emission x-ray absorptiometry, or DEXA scanning. The most important areas to scan are the lumbar spine and hips. Screening examinations measuring more distal bones such as the heel (calcaneus) or radius are less reliable indicators of axial bone loss. Loss of bone mineral density is a continuing process, and levels of loss are defined by comparing bone density either to young adults or to age-matched normal individuals. Results compared to young adults are presented as T-scores, which are standard deviations above or below the normal. In the case of age-matched controls, values are presented as Z-scores, again with the same units of measurement. T-scores or Z-scores of −1.0 or more (≤1 standard deviation below the norm) indicate osteopenia. T-scores or Z-sores of −2.5 or more (≤2.5 standard deviations below normal) indicate osteoporosis.

It is important to monitor bone density over time to check whether persons are responding to treatment. Because each DEXA scanner has a unique profile, efforts should be made to repeat an individual's DEXA scan on the same machine if possible.

If decreased bone density is noted, testing should be done to look for secondary causes of this condition. This should include measuring blood levels of 25-hydroxy vitamin D, calcium, phosphorus, thyroid hormones, parathyroid hormone, complete blood count, and kidney function. If there are below-normal levels of vitamin D, loading that individual with 50,000 IU of vitamin D2 (ergocalciferol) daily for 10 days to 2 weeks and then continuing on a lower dose, as noted below, should be considered. An alternative loading regimen is 50,000 IU of vitamin D2 (ergocalciferol) per week for 24 weeks.

Multiple treatments can be initiated, depending on the severity of the bone density loss and the potential for recovery. Once decreased bone mineral density is diagnosed, treatment is indicated, with repeat DEXA scans every 1 to 2 years. The most commonly used treatments are shown in Table 6.1. Use of biphosphonates, the most common drugs used to treat low bone density, can be associated with complications, such as osteonecrosis of the jaw, atrial fibrillation, and severe muscle pain. Caution is advised in using these agents in persons with dental implants or those with cardiac disease.

Table 6.1 Treatment of Decreased Bone Mineral Density

Clinical Status of the Patient	Severity of Bone Loss	Treatment
Generally ambulatory but treated with recurring steroids or is postmenopausal	Osteopenia (T- or Z-scores ≥−1.0)	1. Encourage weight bearing (prolonged walking, running, weight training). 2. Supplemental calcium citrate, 500 to 600 mg 2 or 3 times a day with food 3. Supplemental vitamin D (at least 1,000 IU per day), after loading, if needed, with vitamin D2, as noted above
	Osteoporosis (T- or Z scores ≥−2.5)	As above, but with the addition of either a bisphosphonate or hormonal replacement, such as raloxifene or parathyroid hormone

Table 6.1 *continued*

Clinical Status of the Patient	Severity of Bone Loss	Treatment
Ambulatory, but limited, with need for either assistive devices or lower-extremity braces	Osteopenia (T- or Z-scores ≥−1.0)	1. Encourage as much walking and weight bearing as possible. 2. Weight training, especially of the lower extremities 3. Supplemental calcium citrate, 500 to 600 mg 2 or 3 times a day with food 4. Supplemental vitamin D (at least 1,000 IU per day), after loading, if needed, with vitamin D2, as noted above
	Osteoporosis (T- or Z scores ≥−2.5)	As above, but with the addition of either a bisphosphonate or hormonal replacement, such as raloxifene or parathyroid hormone
Very limited ambulation or inability to ambulate or even bear weight	Osteopenia (T- or Z-scores ≥−1.0)	1. Supplemental calcium citrate, 500 to 600 mg 2 or 3 times a day with food 2. Supplemental vitamin D (at least 1,000 IU per day), after loading, if needed, with vitamin D2, as noted above 3. Encourage standing as much as possible. 4. If independent standing is not possible, use a standing frame to allow weight bearing at least once per day, as long as tolerated.
	Osteoporosis (T- or Z scores ≥−2.5)	As above but with the addition of either a bisphosphonate or hormonal replacement, such as ralosifene, teriparatide[4] or parathyroid hormone

Sleep Apnea and Other Altered Sleep Patterns

Sleep disturbances are common in persons with MS.[5–11] There are multiple reasons for this. These include increased weight gain as physical activity declines, nocturnal spasms, myoclonus, periodic limb movements, nocturia, MS-related medications, and mood disturbances, such as anxiety and depression. As expected, lack of sleep can contribute greatly to the fatigue that already is an integral symptom of MS.

Inquiring about sleep patterns should be part of any history obtained from persons with MS. Often the causes of poor sleep will be apparent. At other times a formal sleep study will be needed to arrive at a diagnosis and treat accordingly. Avoiding caffeine or other stimulants at night should always be a first approach, as should avoiding marked fluctuations in day–night cycles, avoiding long daytime naps, and practicing "sleep hygiene" (http://www.umm.edu/sleep/sleep_hyg.htm). Some approaches to the management of altered sleep patterns are shown in Table 6.2.

Table 6.2 Approaches to Management of Altered Sleep Patterns

Symptom	Possible Causes	Treatment
Restlessness, choking, loud snoring	Possible obstructive sleep apnea, especially in overweight individuals	Polysomnography to diagnose, followed by use of mouth splints, palatal surgery, or CPAP to relieve the obstruction. Weight loss should also be encouraged.
Early morning awakening	1. Anxiety or depression 2. Excessive daytime sleeping with partial reversal of day-night cycle	1. Use of anxiolytics, such as lorazepam or alprazolam, or use of sedating anti-depressants, such as paroxetine 2. Minimizing daytime sleeping and encourage keeping a regular day/night schedule
Insomnia	1. Anxiety or depression 2. Stimulating medications	1. Use of anxiolytics, such as lorazepam or alprazolam, or use of sedating antidepressants, such as paroxetine, trazodone, or amitriptyline. Some of the newer, non-benzodiazepine soporifics such as zolpidem, zaleplon, eszopidone, and ramelteon, are also of value.[11] 2. Avoiding caffeine or stimulating medications such as modafinil, amantadine, bupropion, or venlafaxine. 3. Practice good sleep hygiene. 4. Maintain a regular day/night cycle.
Intrusive leg movements	1. Nocturnal myoclonus* 2. Restless legs syndrome (RLS)** 3. Spasticity or painful cramping ("charley horses")	1. Clonazepam or another benzodiazepine is a first choice. 2. Pramipexole, or other dopamine agonist 3. Stretching and adequate calcium and magnesium intake; baclofen, tizanidine, or a benzodiazepine, such as diazepam
Nocturia	Either a small, spastic bladder or a large atonic bladder, with incomplete emptying	1. Bladder ultrasound to determine postvoiding residual 2. For small, spastic bladders, use an anticholinergic, such as oxybutynin, tolterodine, solifenacin, trospium, or darifenacin. 3. For large, atonic bladders, use an alpha-adrenergic blocker, such as tamsulosin, alfuzosin, or doxazosin. 4. Avoid beverages containing caffeine or alcohol as both are bladder irritants.

* Nocturnal myoclonus is the occurrence of *involuntary* lower extremity movements, often noted upon initially lying down, but occurring at any time during sleep.

** RLS is characterized by an uncontrollable urge to *voluntarily* move one's legs and is treated differently from myoclonus.

Mood Disturbances

Mood disturbances are another very common comorbidity in persons with MS.[12–16] Disturbances range from depression, to anxiety, to stress, to panic attacks, and any combination of these disorders. Even though mood disturbances should be expected in persons diagnosed with a chronic, potentially disabling disease, the diagnosis and treatment of such disturbances are frequently overlooked. Reasons are multiple, but perhaps most often it is a failure to recognize the pleomorphic manifestations of these changes. At times an individual will admit to depression or anxiety. More often, he or she will deny feeling depressed but will acknowledge the symptoms of mood disturbances, such as insomnia, early morning awakening, loss of appetite or overeating, excessive alcohol intake, irritability and easy angering, lack of conation, anhedonia or inability to feel joy or happiness, inability to concentrate or multitask, difficulties with short-term memory, loss of libido and difficulties with sexual arousal, and fatigue. Some of these difficulties can be a direct result of the disease process, such as cognitive impairment, fatigue, and sexual difficulties. Correlations with other features of that person's difficulties and disabilities may allow differentiation. For example, the presence of bowel and bladder difficulties would suggest that sexual dysfunction may be related to spinal cord disease, while the presence of large lesion loads on MRI, with associated atrophy, would suggest that cognitive difficulties are related, at least in part, to structural changes and not entirely to mood.

Treatment of the mood alterations associated with MS varies with the symptoms. Selective serotonin reuptake inhibitors (SSRIs) are a staple of the treatment for depression. More sedating drugs such as paroxetine or a tricyclic antidepressant can be used for persons with anxiety, emotional lability, and insomnia, and venlafaxine or bupropion can be used for persons with lack of energy or lack of conation. Anxiety and stress are similarly managed with anxiolytics such as lorazepam, alprazolam, or buspirone. I routinely treat mood alterations in my practice using the lowest possible doses and choosing the drug based on the characteristics (anxiety, emotional lability, loss of conation, insomnia, lack of concentration) of that individual's difficulties. Responses to a particular antidepressant and anxiolytic, in terms of both efficacy and side effects, vary greatly among individuals, and the "failure" of one drug should not dissuade one from trying other, albeit similar agents.

Suicide rates in persons with MS are higher than those of the general population and persons with more severe mood alterations, especially those with suicidal thoughts, should be immediately referred for psychiatric evaluation and counseling. Inquiring about suicidal ideation should be part of any evaluation of depression in persons with MS.

Urinary Tract and Other Infections

For multiple reasons infections, especially urinary tract infections (UTIs), are more common in persons with MS than in the general population.[17,18]

An important cause of UTIs is incomplete bladder emptying and the use of indwelling catheters.[19,20] Bladder sensation is often impaired, leading to infrequent voiding and inability to feel the discomforts of a UTI. Patients may choose to dehydrate themselves to avoid urinary frequency and loss of control, and women with decreased vaginal and clitoral sensation may need prolonged and vigorous stimulation during sexual intercourse, increasing the likelihood of introducing bacteria into the urethra. Pressure sores and abscesses can occur in more debilitated individuals with MS, as can aspiration pneumonia. Sinus infections also are common in persons with MS, perhaps due to the anticholinergic, mucosal-drying properties of many of the medications used to treat MS symptoms, such as used for bladder dysfunction.

Any infectious process can make the symptoms of MS worse. Such worsening is considered a "pseudo-exacerbation" and not the result of a new, inflammatory CNS process. Symptoms usually resolve with treatment of the infection; the use of steroids, which may decrease the individual's ability to fight the infection, should be avoided. Because of the delicate balance between function and dysfunction in the CNS of persons with MS, even very mild, almost unobtrusive, infections can cause significant changes in symptoms and signs. Thus, any person being evaluated for an MS relapse should first have a screening, by history, examination, and if appropriate laboratory studies, for infection, especially a UTI.

UTIs are among the most common infections seen in persons with MS.[17,18] If the classic symptoms of a UTI are present—increased urinary frequency and urgency, altered urine color and odor, dysuria, and lower abdominal pain—the diagnosis can easily be made. All too often, however, because of decreased bladder sensations, these symptoms are lacking, and other manifestations are present. Most commonly these include worsening of lower extremity spasticity and weakness, increased fatigue, increased numbness and tingling or tremors, or increased imbalance. In other words, either existing neurologic symptoms are worsened, or previous neurologic symptoms reappear. This being the case, in our practice we routinely obtain a urinalysis and if appropriate a urine culture in persons who have a sudden change in their neurologic symptoms. About one third of the time there will be a cryptic UTI, which, when treated, results in resolution of symptoms.[17]

As will be noted in Chapter 7, infections, especially viral infections, predispose to the appearance of true MS exacerbations.[21] Such relapses usually occur several weeks after recovery from the infection. If clinically indicated, standard relapse treatment is warranted.

Sexual Dysfunction

Because of discomfort about the subject on the part of the patient or the medical provider, sexual function is one of the most frequently overlooked comorbidities associated with MS.[22–27] As noted in the section on mood alterations, persons with MS frequently have difficulties with sexual function. The drugs used to treat such mood alterations, in particular SSRI antidepressants, also can have a profound effect in terms of decreasing libido and ease of arousal. While both mood and medication can contribute to altered sexual function, spinal cord dysfunction can also be a major contributor, with difficulty with arousal, insufficient lubrication, and inability to achieve orgasm, or maintain erections. Treatments will, as always, vary with the difficulties.

In women, increasing vaginal and clitoral stimulation is often successful. The two methods recommended in my practice are vibrators and changes in position. Multiple variations of vibrators are now available, including ones that fit on the erect penis, and only imagination and the partner's willingness are limiting. Changing position also is effective, such as the woman assuming the top position, allowing her more freedom to stimulate herself. Multiple water-soluble lubricants are available to help with this issue, although patients should be cautioned not to use petroleum-based lubricants.

Lack of penile sensation is common in men with MS, with associated erectile dysfunction. Vasodilating agents such as sildenafil, tadalafil, and vardenafil are of value.[24] Referral to a urologist specializing in male sexual dysfunction is recommended if vacuum pumps, penile rings, prostaglandin pellets or injections, or penile prostheses are needed.

Skin Lesions

The most common skin lesions seen in persons with MS result from the use of injectable disease-modifying therapies.[28–31] These can range from mild redness and swelling to necrosis, infection, and abscess (Table 6.3). Reactions can be minimized by warming the medications to room temperature before injection, using shorter needles and decreasing injection depth in thin persons, warming the injection sites with compresses before injection (though some patients prefer cooling the injection sites), using slower manual injections rather than automatic injectors, being as clean as possible (with handwashing, preparing the skin with alcohol before injection, and allowing the alcohol to dry completely before injecting), and assiduously avoiding injections into muscle or intradermally. Muscle injections of the subcutaneously injected drugs, in particular glatiramer acetate, can be very painful, with significant ecchymosis at those sites. Subcutaneous lipoatrophy and fibrosis can also be seen in persons injecting glatiramer acetate for extended periods. This appears to be specific to certain individuals, as others who have taken this medication for years do not have such responses. Nevertheless, the presence of lipoatrophy and fibrosis, while not serious, can make injections very difficult due to inability to penetrate the fibrotic areas. Injecting into less accessible regions may be the only alternative.

Patients with MS who lose their ability to ambulate and spend most of their time sitting in wheelchairs or recliners or in bed are especially liable to get skin lesions in the form of pressure sores over the sacrum or buttocks, or fungal infections of skin creases. Pressure sores can become sources of major disability, and prevention is the best approach. Proper diet to ensure adequate protein intake to maintain tissue integrity is essential, especially

Table 6.3 Skin Lesions Induced by Injectable Disease-Modifying Therapies

Drug	Skin Changes	Treatment
Glatiramer acetate	1. *Immediate*: Burning, itching, redness, pain, and swelling, lasting for minutes to hours	1a. Inject drug at room temperature, or even at body temperature, by holding the solution in the hand or under an armpit for 5 minutes.
		1b. Pretreat the skin with either warm or cold compresses for 30 to 60 seconds.
		1c. Clean skin with alcohol, but inject only after the alcohol has totally evaporated.
		1d. Slow injections by hand are preferred by some over the rapid injection noted with the spring-loaded injector.
		1e. Apply an antihistamine cream or ointment to the injection site (e.g., diphenhydramine).
		1f. Assiduously avoid injecting into muscle. Very painful and can cause marked ecchymosis. In areas with little subcutaneous tissue, use a shorter needle or decrease depth setting of the automatic injector.
	2. *Intermediate and Delayed*: Induration, lipoatrophy, more diffuse subcutaneous fibrosis, abscess, and necrosis	2. Most "lumps" at injection sites will gradually decrease over time. Massaging the "lumps" can help.
		2b. No treatment for lipoatrophy or the generalized skin fibrosis
		2c. Prevention of abscesses is best, with careful handwashing and skin cleansing with alcohol.
Subcutaneous beta-interferons	1. *Immediate*: Similar skin reactions as with glatiramer acetate	1. Reactions due to local release of cytokines. Treatment similar to that noted with glatiramer acetate.
	2. *Intermediate and Delayed*: Induration, abscess, and necrosis. Lower incidence of lipoatrophy and skin fibrosis than with glatiramer acetate.	2. Necrosis may be due to infection but also can result from cytokine release. Nevertheless, careful handwashing and skin preparation with alcohol rub should be done.
Intramuscular beta-interferon	1. *Immediate*: Minor to none	
	2. *Intermediate and Delayed*: Uncommon, but occasional deep abscesses can form.	1. As noted above, prevention of abscesses is best, with careful handwashing and skin cleansing with alcohol.

in persons with difficulties chewing and swallowing. Adequate cushions and seating supports for wheelchairs also are of great importance. There are specialized wheelchair seating clinics that can measure areas of greatest pressure and design cushions and supports specific to an individual. If individualization of seating is not available, special wheelchair cushions such as the Roho® cushion, Gel-foam, or eggcrate foam cushions can be used. Special mattress padding is of great value for bedbound individuals, such as Gel-foam, eggcrate foam, or alternating air pressure pads. Heel protectors also should be considered, both for persons confined to wheelchairs and bed-bound patients.

Many persons with MS are overweight due to their inability to move about and exercise, or have associated difficulties with showering and bathing and loss of bladder and bowel control. As a result, the risks of intertrigo, or irritation and infection of skin folds in the groin and axillae, under breasts, or under abdominal folds, is increased. Again, prevention is best, with good hygiene and keeping such areas dry and exposed to air, if possible. Light, white, cotton cloth can be placed between skin folds to absorb moisture. If intertrigo develops, compresses with Burow's solution 1:40, dilute vinegar, or wet tea bags may be of value, but these areas must then be dried carefully. If fungal infections supervene, antimycotic creams or ointments containing miconazole or clotrimazole should be considered, combined with short-term use of low-dose topical steroids.

Joint Dysfunction

Joint dysfunction, with pain, hyperextension, and contractures, occurs frequently in persons with MS.[32] Limb weakness or spasticity, especially involving the lower extremities, results in altered walking dynamics, with greatly increased stresses on the knees, ankles, and lower back. As a result, "wear and tear" of these areas increases with increased risk of osteoarthritis and ligamentous injury. Weight gain is also a contributing factor as mobility decreases. With upper extremity weakness and spasticity, reduced movements can result in the development of finger contractures and "frozen" shoulders and elbows. Again, prevention is the best approach.

The staples of therapy are exercising muscles to maintain optimal strength and weight; daily range of motion and stretching; individualized bracing of weakened joints, such as ankle–foot orthoses (AFOs); training in the proper use of canes, walkers, and other assistive devices; and use of anti-inflammatory and analgesic medications to allow greater mobility. The expertise of a physiatrist, trained physical therapists, occupational therapists, orthotists, and exercise physiologists is of major importance, and they should be involved whenever possible.

Obesity

As with many other chronic illnesses in which decreased mobility is a component, persons with MS have a high rate of obesity.[33] While prevention is the best approach, for many persons that is not possible. Some individuals have been overweight for years, with multiple attempts to lose weight with fad diets, only to quickly regain it when off diet. Discouragement and resignation are common, but strong and repeated encouragement, emphasizing improving mobility, balance, energy, and endurance, should be repeatedly provided. Most patients are already well aware of the benefits of weight loss in regards to their MS, as well as for reducing the risk of hypertension, diabetes mellitus, and heart disease. The main issues are breaking old habits and having the motivation to do so. Referral to a dietitian experienced in working with persons with neurologic difficulties can be a valuable option.

Some patients may choose to have bariatric surgery. This certainly is effective, but the complication rates with some of the procedures are considerable and short-term worsening of MS symptoms may result.[34] With more complex bypass procedures long-term dietary management may be needed, possibly complicating use of the multiple oral medications that may be needed for symptom management. These issues should be discussed in detail before surgery.

References

1. Cosman F, Nieves J, Komar L, et al. Fracture history and bone loss in patients with MS. Neurology. 1998;51:1161–1165.

2. Ozgocmen S, Bulut S, Ilhan N, et al. Vitamin D deficiency and reduced bone mineral density in multiple sclerosis: effect of ambulatory status and functional capacity. J Bone Miner Metab. 2005;23:309–313.

3. Weinstock-Guttman B, Gallagher E, Baier M, et al. Risk of bone loss in men with multiple sclerosis. Mult Scler. 2004;10:170–175.

4. Bilezikian JP. Combination anabolic and antiresorptive therapy for osteoporosis: opening the anabolic window. Curr Osteoporos Rep. 2008;6:24–30.

5. Kaynak H, Altintas A, Kaynak D, et al. Fatigue and sleep disturbance in multiple sclerosis. Eur J Neurol. 2006;13:1333–1339.

6. Manconi M, Fabbrini M, Bonanni E, et al. High prevalence of restless legs syndrome in multiple sclerosis. Eur J Neurol. 2007;14:534–539.

7. Merlino G, Fratticci L, Lenchig C, et al. Prevalence of 'poor sleep' among patients with multiple sclerosis: an independent predictor of mental and physical status. Sleep Med. 2008 Jan. 18 [E-pub before print].

8. Merlino G, Valente M, Serafini A, Gigli GL. Restless legs syndrome: diagnosis, epidemiology, classification and consequences. Neurol Sci. 2007;28(Suppl 1):S37–46.

9. Stanton BR, Barnes F, Silber E. Sleep and fatigue in multiple sclerosis. Mult Scler. 2006;12:481–486.

10. Tachibana N, Howard RS, Hirsch NP, et al. Sleep problems in multiple sclerosis. Eur Neurol. 1994;34:320–323.

11. Ramakrishnan K, Scheid DC. Treatment options for insomnia. Am Fam Physician. 2007;76:517–526.

12. Beal CC, Stuifbergen AK, Brown A. Depression in multiple sclerosis: a longitudinal analysis. Arch Psychiatr Nurs. 2007;21:181–191.

13. Beiske AG, Svensson E, Sandanger I, et al. Depression and anxiety amongst multiple sclerosis patients. Eur J Neurol. 2008;15:239–245.

14. Chwastiak LA, Ehde DM. Psychiatric issues in multiple sclerosis. Psychiatr Clin North Am. 2007;30:803–817.

15. Mohr DC, Hart SL, Julian L, Tasch ES. Screening for depression among patients with multiple sclerosis: two questions may be enough. *Mult Scler.* 2007;13:215–219.

16. Wilken JA, Sullivan C. Recognizing and treating common psychiatric disorders in multiple sclerosis. *Neurologist.* 2007;13:343–354.

17. Edlich RF, Westwater JJ, Lombardi SA, et al. Multiple sclerosis and asymptomatic urinary tract infection. *J Emerg Med.* 1990;8:25–28.

18. Foxman B. Epidemiology of urinary tract infections: incidence, morbidity, and economic costs. *Dis Mon.* 2003;49:53–70.

19. Rashid TM, Hollander JB. Multiple sclerosis and the neurogenic bladder. *Phys Med Rehabil Clin North Am.* 1998;9:615–629.

20. Gallien P, Robineau S, Nicolas B, et al. Vesicourethral dysfunction and urodynamic findings in multiple sclerosis: a study of 149 cases. *Arch Phys Med Rehabil.* 1998;79:255–257.

21. Buljevac D, Flach HZ, Hop WC, et al. Prospective study on the relationship between infections and multiple sclerosis exacerbations. *Brain.* 2002;125:952–960.

22. Bitzer J, Platano G, Tschudin S, Alder J. Sexual counseling for women in the context of physical diseases: a teaching model for physicians. *J Sex Med.* 2007;4:29–37.

23. Gruenwald I, Vardi Y, Gartman I, et al. Sexual dysfunction in females with multiple sclerosis: quantitative sensory testing. *Mult Scler.* 2007;13:95–105.

24. Landtblom AM. Treatment of erectile dysfunction in multiple sclerosis. *Expert Rev Neurother.* 2006;6:931–935.

25. Moore LA. Intimacy and multiple sclerosis. *Nurs Clin North Am.* 2007;42:605–619.

26. Nortvedt MW, Riise T, Frugard J, et al. Prevalence of bladder, bowel and sexual problems among multiple sclerosis patients two to five years after diagnosis. *Mult Scler.* 2007;13:106–112.

27. Tzortzis V, Skriapas K, Hadjigeorgiou G, et al. Sexual dysfunction in newly diagnosed multiple sclerosis women. *Mult Scler.* 2008 Jan. 31 [E-pub ahead of print].

28. Frohman EM, Brannon K, Alexander S, et al. Disease-modifying agent–related skin reactions in multiple sclerosis: prevention, assessment, and management. *Mult Scler.* 2004;10:302–307.

29. Arrue I, Saiz A, Ortiz-Romero PL, Rodriguez-Peralto JL. Lupus-like reaction to interferon at the injection site: report of five cases. *J Cutan Pathol.* 2007;34(Suppl 1):18–21.

30. Bosca I, Bosca M, Belenguer A, et al. Necrotising cutaneous lesions as a side effect of glatiramer acetate. *J Neurol.* 2006;253:1370–1371.

31. Edgar CM, Brunet DG, Fenton P, et al. Lipoatrophy in patients with multiple sclerosis on glatiramer acetate. *Can J Neurol Sci.* 2004;31:58–63.

32. DeLisa JA, Hammond MC, Mikulic MA, Miller RM. Multiple sclerosis: Part I. Common physical disabilities and rehabilitation. *Am Fam Physician.* 1985;32:157–163.

33. Payne A. Nutrition and diet in the clinical management of multiple sclerosis. *J Hum Nutr Diet.* 2001;14:349–357.

34. Flanagan L, Jr. Is bariatric surgery effective in the treatment of the neurological motor deficit syndromes? *Obes Surg.* 1997;7:420–423.

Chapter 7

Relapses of Multiple Sclerosis and Their Treatment

What Constitutes a Relapse?

Biologically, an MS relapse (flare, exacerbation, attack) is defined as a clinical worsening due to a new or expanding area of CNS inflammation. Clinically, the change in neurologic symptoms and signs should persist for more than 48 hours. Only two conditions have been persuasively linked to an increased risk of relapses. These are the period 2 to 6 months postpartum, when a woman's immune system readjusts to normal,[1–4] and the period 1 to 5 weeks following an infection, usually a viral infection.[5,6] The reason for the latter phenomenon is not known but is believed to result from a stimulation of the immune system following its response to the infectious agent.[7]

Pseudo-exacerbations

Making the diagnosis of an MS relapse can be difficult. Many factors can contribute to a worsening of symptoms and signs in persons with MS that are not the result of new CNS inflammation. Worsening of signs and symptoms resulting from non–MS-related disease processes is called a "pseudo-relapse" or "pseudo-exacerbation." These phenomena should always be considered before diagnosing a true MS attack. Some of the most common and important non-MS causes of increased symptoms and signs are noted in Table 7.1.

Conventional Relapse Treatments

Once the above factors have been evaluated and eliminated, the exact nature of the relapse needs to be determined in terms of its severity and its effect on the individual's functioning. Since relapses can resolve on their own, at times without residua, the decision to treat should be made on the basis of the severity of symptoms, their duration, and if applicable the previous pattern of relapses in that individual. In other words, if the main manifestation of a person's MS is recurring bouts of mild paresthesias, unaccompanied by changes in the physical examination or functioning,

Table 7.1 Non–MS-Related Causes of Worsening Signs or Symptoms (Pseudo-exacerbations)

Causes	Management
Infection: One of most common, and often overlooked, causes of MS worsening. The infection can be of a low grade and may or may not be associated with fever. Urinary tract infections are most common; because of decreased bladder sensation often the classic symptoms of a UTI are not present.[8]	1. Thorough history with emphasis on urinary tract, upper respiratory tract, sinus, skin, and teeth. 2. Obtain a CBC and UA/UC if there is any uncertainty, and treat any infection as appropriate. Corticosteroids need not be administered.
Increased core temperature: Can occur with exercise, hot baths or showers, dehydration, increases in ambient temperature, and sepsis	1. If symptoms are short-lived and resolve with cooling down (Uthoff's phenomenon), reassure the patient that the event was benign. 2. If elevated ambient temperatures are the cause, advise the patient to wear a light-colored brimmed hat in the sun, drink cool liquids, and wear a cooling neck collar. Patients who need to be outside can put their feet in a tub of cool water. 3. If fever is believed to be the cause, evaluate and treat the cause of the presumed infection.
Stress, depression, and fatigue: Poor sleeping habits often accompany depression and increased stress levels, resulting in increased weakness and worsening of previous symptoms.[9,10]	1. If stress is the major factor, counseling and antidepressant or anti-anxiety medications can help. 2. Treating non-stress-related fatigue with treatment of sleep disorders (see Chapter 6) and with energy-increasing medications such as modafinil or amantadine can be considered. 3. Regular exercise also can significantly relieve these symptoms and should be encouraged.

with spontaneous resolution to baseline, treatment may not be needed. Similarly, administering steroids to a person who had a relapse weeks to months previously, in an effort to reduce residual disability, may not be effective. On the other hand, a person with recurring bouts of major motor, cerebellar, or sensory changes, with residua from previous attacks, should be treated aggressively at the onset of a relapse, once confounding issues such as infection have been excluded.

The intent of relapse treatment is to shorten the duration of a relapse and, by reducing inflammation, to allow better healing with less residua. The former can usually be achieved, but the latter is uncertain. The most common category of drugs used to treat MS relapses is the corticosteroids.[11] Table 7.2 lists the most commonly used steroids, their major side effects, treatment of the side effects, and protocols for administration. As noted below, drugs can be administered either orally or intravenously; clinical benefits and side effects with either route are similar. While large numbers

Table 7.2 Treatment of MS Relapses With Corticosteroids

Drug	Route of Administration	Treatment Protocol
Methylprednisolone	Oral or IV	*Oral*: 1,000 mg in 2 or 3 divided doses per day for 3 to 7 days. Length of treatment depends on the severity of the attack and patient's tolerance and response. *IV*: 1c000 mg in 100 cc of 5% dextrose solution, administered slowly over 90 to 120 minutes. Speed of infusion should be slowed if blood pressure or heart rate rises. Careful monitoring of vital signs is necessary during the initial infusion, and thereafter if indicated by the initial response.
Prednisone or presdnisolone	Oral	Because of differences in equivalency compared to methylprednisolone, 1,250 mg of drug is administered daily for 3 to 7 days; duration varies with the severity of the attack and the patient's response.
Dexamethasone	Oral or IV	Because of differences in equivalency compared to methylprednisolone, 160 mg of this drug is administered daily for 3 to 7 days; duration varies with the severity of the attack and the patient's response.
Steroid-tapering medications, (methylprednisolone or prednisone)	Oral	Tapering is usually recommended following treatment with high-dose oral or IV steroids for more than 3 to 5 days, especially in patients with a history of withdrawal symptoms. Starting doses of tapering steroids range from 48 mg/day for methylprednisolone to 60 mg/day for prednisone, tapering over 6 to 14 days, depending on the patient's response.

of pills may be needed to achieve doses equivalent to the intravenous route, gastric side effects are usually not noted.[12] Tapering off high doses of corticosteroids may be necessary to avoid withdrawal symptoms, especially when treatment duration is more than 3 days.

Because of the frequency of certain side effects with administration of steroids, especially high-dose steroids, we routinely advise a low-salt, high-potassium diet while on steroids, and we preemptively prescribe a soporific and an H2 blocker or proton pump inhibitor to prevent insomnia and abdominal discomfort, respectively (Table 7.3). The frequency of insomnia and abdominal discomfort with steroids appears to be the same for both intravenous and oral treatment protocols.

Table 7.3 Corticosteroid Side Effects and Their Management

Possible Side Effects	Treatment of Side Effects
Insomnia	Use soporifics such as lorazepam, temazepam, zolpidem. Because of the frequency of this side effect we preemptively prescribe one of these drugs.
Abdominal discomfort, bloating, acid reflux	H2 blockers or proton pump inhibitors. Because of the frequency of this side effect we preemptively prescribe one of these drugs.
Fluid retention	Low-salt, high-potassium diet. Rarely is a diuretic needed.
Mood changes (anxiety, depression, or emotional lability)	If severe enough to disrupt function, lithium carbonate, 300 mg bid, should be started, 1 to 2 days before onset of treatment and during steroid taper. Lorazepam or aprazaolam for anxiety is also very effective.
Red face	No treatment is needed, just reassurance that this will subside.
Acne	Usually no treatment is needed as this too will clear up.
Blurred vision and trouble focusing	Usually due to mild corneal edema. No treatment is needed, as this will resolve.
Elevated blood sugar levels	In diabetics, additional doses of insulin may be needed.
Elevated blood pressure and heart rate	Usually occurs during the IV infusion of steroids. Slowing the rate of infusion will often suffice.
Muscle and joint soreness and aching, usually after stopping the drug or during the tapering phase of treatment. Can be associated with worsening of MS symptoms too.	Most often noted after more prolonged high-dose steroid treatment. Slow the rate of steroid taper or treat with ibuprofen, acetaminophen, or naproxen. If there is persistent joint pain, especially hip pain, screen for the presence of aseptic necrosis of the head of the femur with an MRI of the hip. If aseptic necrosis of the head of the femur is present, stop steroids and refer to an orthopedist for evaluation.
Hives, shortness of breath, facial swelling	Allergic reactions to steroids can occur, though they are uncommon. Stop treatment and administer either antihistamines or epinephrine as indicated.
Chest pain, chest pressure, or other signs of cardiac dysfunction	Persons with antecedent heart disease or those at high risk for ischemic heart disease can have increasing symptoms and even infarctions during IV administration of high-dose steroids.[13,14] Infusions should be stopped and appropriate monitoring and treatment initiated.

Unconventional Relapse Treatments

While an additional course of steroids is always an option in persons with an insufficient response to an initial pulse, other treatment options can be considered in individuals with severe attacks refractory to even multiple courses of steroids. The two most often considered are intravenous IgG and plasmapheresis.

IV IgG

The value of treatment with IV IgG for acute relapses is controversial.[15] Some small clinical trials have shown benefit, but larger trials have not. Because of these conflicting data, IV IgG should be considered a second-line therapy. As is always the case with larger clinical trials, variations in response among individuals are obscured. Thus, some individuals with MS may respond better to IV IgG than to high-dose steroids. The dosage and duration of treatment vary greatly among clinical trials.[15]

Plasmapheresis

One single-center, double-blind, placebo-controlled trial showed, in a subgroup of patients with severe relapses of MS refractory to treatment with high-dose corticosteroids, that a course of plasmapheresis resulted in significant short-term improvement.[16] Relapses eventually recurred, but in some individuals improvements following plasmapheresis were dramatic. Selecting patients for treatment with plasmapheresis is difficult. Preliminary data suggest that patients with type 2 immunopathologic changes on brain biopsy (that is, those showing the presence of antibodies at sites of demyelination) are the best responders.[17] Since biopsies are not generally available on most MS patients and there are no other markers for this pattern of demyelination, empirical treatment is the only option. Patients with neuromyelitis optica (Devic's disease), who often have antibodies to the CNS protein aquaporin 4 and who, at autopsy, have large amounts of antibodies and complement components present at sites of myelin destruction, also can respond well in the short term to plasmapheresis (see Chapter 3).

There is no standard protocol for plasmapheresis, but five 1.5 plasma-volume exchanges over 10 days, with replacement of volume with human serum albumin, has been used with good effect. The monoclonal antibody rituximab, directed against the B-cell protein CD20, has been used in small clinical trials of neuromyelitis optica to selectively reduce B cells with some success.[18] However, such use is "off label" and should be considered experimental at this time.

Relapse Prevention

As noted above, only two conditions are persuasively associated with the appearance of relapses in MS: infections and the immediate postpartum period.

Postinfectious relapses are most common in the 1 to 5 weeks following recovery and are usually not difficult to separate from the "pseudo-exacerbations" occurring during infections. Most relapse-associated infections are viral upper respiratory tract infections. Preventing relapses after infections, especially viral infections, is difficult. However, annual vaccination of MS patients with flu vaccine should be strongly encouraged in those not allergic to vaccine components. At present there are no persuasive data showing that vaccination results in increased MS-related disease activity.[19–21]

Low-grade chronic infections may play a role in increasing the general level of immune activity in the host. Treatment of low-grade infections, such as sinus infections, gingivitis, and periodontal disease, should be encouraged.

In view of an increased risk of an MS relapse in the 2- to 6-month postpartum period, and the diathesis of some women with MS to have this as a pattern of their illness, some MS neurologists choose to preemptively treat such individuals with either IV steroids or IV IgG during the immediate postpartum period, and then monthly for up to 6 months. Results of small clinical trials have been inconclusive, with some showing benefit and others not. At this time there are no markers to predict which women are at particular risk for relapses.[1] Breastfeeding does not appear to have a protective effect.[22] Reassuringly, several studies failed to show long-term adverse effects on the course of MS following postpartum relapses.[4,23,24] At this time, preemptive treatment of relapses should be considered an unproven treatment option.

References

1. Vukusic S, Hutchinson M, Hours M, et al. Pregnancy and multiple sclerosis (the PRIMS study): clinical predictors of post-partum relapse. *Brain*. 2004; 127:1353–1360.

2. Airas L, Saraste M, Rinta S, et al. Immunoregulatory factors in multiple sclerosis patients during and after pregnancy: relevance of natural killer cells. *Clin Exp Immunol*. 2008;151:235–243.

3. Airas L, Nikula T, Huang YH, et al. Postpartum-activation of multiple sclerosis is associated with down-regulation of tolerogenic HLA-G. *J Neuroimmunol*. 2007;187:205–211.

4. Damek DM, Shuster EA. Pregnancy and multiple sclerosis. *Mayo Clin Proc*. 1997;72:977–989.

5. Buljevac D, Flach HZ, Hop WC, et al. Prospective study on the relationship between infections and multiple sclerosis exacerbations. *Brain*. 2002;125:952–960.

6. Panitch HS. Influence of infection on exacerbations of multiple sclerosis. *Ann Neurol*. 1994;36(Suppl):S25–28.

7. Correale J, Fiol M, Gilmore W. The risk of relapses in multiple sclerosis during systemic infections. *Neurology*. 2006;67:652–659.

8. Edlich RF, Westwater JJ, Lombardi SA, et al. Multiple sclerosis and asymptomatic urinary tract infection. *J Emerg Med*. 1990;8:25–28.

9. Golan D, Somer E, Dishon S, et al. Impact of exposure to war stress on exacerbations of multiple sclerosis. *Ann Neurol*. 2008 June 28 [E-pub before print].

10. Mohr DC. Stress and multiple sclerosis. *J Neurol*. 2007;254 Suppl 2:II65–68.

11. Frohman EM, Shah A, Eggenberger E, et al. Corticosteroids for multiple sclerosis: I. Application for treating exacerbations. *Neurotherapeutics*. 2007;4:618–626.

12. Metz LM, Sabuda D, Hilsden RJ, et al. Gastric tolerance of high-dose pulse oral prednisone in multiple sclerosis. *Neurology*. 1999;53:2093–2096.

13. Cerisier A, Dacosta A, Dubois F, et al. [Myocardial infarction following rapid perfusion of corticoids]. *Arch Mal Coeur Vaiss*. 1995;88:521–523.

14. Smith RS, Warren DJ. Effects of high-dose intravenous methylprednisolone on circulation in humans. *Transplantation*. 1983;35:349–351.

15. Soelberg Sorensen P. Intravenous polyclonal human immunoglobulins in multiple sclerosis. *Neurodegener Dis*. 2008;5:8–15.

16. Weinshenker BG, O'Brien PC, Petterson TM, et al. A randomized trial of plasma exchange in acute central nervous system inflammatory demyelinating disease. *Ann Neurol*. 1999;46:878–886.

17. Lucchinetti CF, Bruck W, Lassmann H. Evidence for pathogenic heterogeneity in multiple sclerosis. *Ann Neurol*. 2004;56:308.

18. Cree BA, Lamb S, Morgan K, et al. An open label study of the effects of rituximab in neuromyelitis optica. *Neurology*. 2005;64:1270–1272.

19. DeStefano F, Verstraeten T, Jackson LA, et al. Vaccinations and risk of central nervous system demyelinating diseases in adults. *Arch Neurol*. 2003;60:504–509.

20. Moriabadi NF, Niewiesk S, Kruse N, et al. Influenza vaccination in MS: absence of T-cell response against white matter proteins. *Neurology*. 2001;56:938–943.

21. Rutschmann OT, McCrory DC, Matchar DB. Immunization and MS: a summary of published evidence and recommendations. *Neurology*. 2002;59:1837–1843.

22. Nelson LM, Franklin GM, Jones MC. Risk of multiple sclerosis exacerbation during pregnancy and breast-feeding. *JAMA*. 1988;259:3441–3443.

23. Houtchens MK. Pregnancy and multiple sclerosis. *Semin Neurol*. 2007; 27:434–441.

24. Runmarker B, Andersen O. Pregnancy is associated with a lower risk of onset and a better prognosis in multiple sclerosis. *Brain*. 1995;118(Pt 1):253–261.

Chapter 8

Long-Term Disease-Modifying Therapies

The introduction in the early 1990s of medications that clearly modified the course of MS revolutionized treatment of the disease. Prior to that time the approach of many neurologists was to intervene at the time of acute relapses and to treat symptoms as they arose, but otherwise it was "diagnose and adios."

One of the initial pivotal observations on disease-modifying therapies in MS was made in 1981 by Dr. Lawrence Jacobs, who noted that intrathecal interferon-beta reduced MS relapses.[1] Twelve years later the first large, double-blind, placebo-controlled trial of interferon-beta was published, and the era of modern therapy for MS began.[2,3] As of this writing six drugs approved by the U.S. Food and Drug Administration (FDA) for the treatment of MS are available in the United States. All of them are anti-inflammatories, but they have a variety of mechanisms of action. Most are approved only for persons with relapsing-remitting MS, with one drug, mitoxantrone,[4] approved for persons with rapidly progressive secondary-progressive MS. Unfortunately, there are no approved drugs available at this time for persons with primary-progressive MS or the more usual gradually progressive secondary-progressive MS.

All of the current disease-modifying therapies require injections—subcutaneous, intramuscular, or intravenous (IV). Oral drugs are used in selected individuals with relapsing-remitting MS, but their use is "off label" and not approved by the FDA for that purpose. Multiple clinical trials are in progress with agents that have potential to be first-line disease-modifying therapies. However, their efficacy must be at least as good as the current drugs, as safe, and as well tolerated. That will take time to ascertain.

Issues with Long-Term Immune-Modulating Therapies

Choosing a Disease-Modifying Therapy

Patients always ask, "What is the best drug for me?" Since I believe MS is a syndrome and not a disease, with multiple potential pathways leading to demyelination and axonal destruction, I cannot easily answer that question.

There are no "bad" disease-modifying therapies on the market, and recent "head-to-head" trials, comparing different disease-modifying therapies, and as of this writing unpublished, suggest that, at least in groups of individuals, high-dose beta-interferons and glatiramer acetate are equivalent. That said, on an individual level there are major differences in how a person's MS responds to the different treatments. In some individuals the response is quite dramatic, with almost complete cessation of disease activity. More commonly there is a reduction in disease activity. Some individuals do not respond at all to a particular drug, and changing treatment is necessary. However, since none of the disease-modifying therapies has an instant effect on disease course, and preexisting lesions will continue to evolve after initiation of disease-modifying therapy, it usually takes 6 to 12 months on a drug to determine an individual's pattern of treatment response (see also Chapter 3).

It is tempting to compare efficacies of the disease-modifying therapies across different clinical trials, but such comparisons are misleading and inaccurate. Outcomes of a trial are dependent on the control groups, and these vary greatly between trials. In addition, entry criteria, the quality of disease monitoring, and primary and secondary outcomes vary considerably between trials, further compromising the validity of cross-trial comparisons.

Ensuring Treatment Adherence and Compliance

Having realistic expectations is a key factor in maintaining long-term adherence to disease-modifying therapies. Since none of the treatments is a cure for the disease, it is essential to emphasize to every patient that continued disease activity may still occur, but ideally the frequency and severity of episodes will be reduced. In addition, repeated emphasis must be placed on the fact that none of the disease-modifying therapies can reverse what has already happened, and thus they will not improve a person's disabilities. Therefore, the statement often heard that "I can't tell any difference in my MS since starting treatment" may actually be an indicator of therapeutic efficacy and should be a sign of encouragement to the patient.

Two other important factors in determining adherence to long-term immune modulating therapies are side effects and costs. Beta-interferons almost always induce flu-like symptoms, which vary in intensity in different individuals. These respond well to over-the-counter medications such as aspirin, ibuprofen, or naproxen and tend to resolve over time. Injection site reactions are an important issue, and again, information regarding the possible occurrence of red, itchy, lumpy injection sites must be discussed at the beginning of treatment with the subcutaneously injected medications (see Chapter 6). Less common consequences of liver, thyroid, bone marrow, and cardiac dysfunction should also be discussed with patients taking beta-interferons, as should the need to monitor for such adverse events.[5] The possibility of systemic reactions and allergic responses should be reviewed with patients receiving glatiramer acetate. For the IV injected medications, the possibility of cardiac dysfunction with heart failure and leukemia must be discussed as hazards of mitoxantrone treatment;[6,7] for natalizumab, the possibility of progressive multifocal leukoencephalopathy, opportunistic infections, liver failure, and melanoma must be reviewed.[8–12]

Cost is an issue in countries without universal health care. In the United States, many MS patients are finding that copayments for their disease-modifying therapies are beyond reach. Several of the pharmaceutical companies and disease advocacy organizations have funds available to help with such copayments.

When Do I Initiate Treatment With Disease-Modifying Therapies?

Treatment with disease-modifying therapies should be initiated as early as possible in all patients with *active* relapsing-remitting MS. What is active relapsing-remitting MS? These are individuals with either recurring clinical attacks or those with continued accumulation of lesions, even asymptomatic ones, on MRI.[13–18] There are data from the early, pivotal, placebo-controlled trials, that patients who delay therapy for 2 years never recover from the disability accumulated during their years on placebo, compared with patients initiating treatment years earlier. Even more important are recent data suggesting that responses to disease-modifying therapies in current patient populations are even greater than those seen in pivotal trials. In the original pivotal trials of the beta-interferons and glatiramer acetate, annualized relapse rate reductions of about 30% were noted. In recent head-to-head studies involving high-dose beta-interferons and glatiramer acetate, relapse rate reductions in the range of 70% to 80% were noted (REGARD and BEYOND trials). As discussed earlier, comparisons between clinical trials for degrees of efficacy cannot be made. However, these levels of relapse rate reduction in the recent trials set a new standard for efficacy that subsequent therapies will need to meet.

As noted in Chapter 3, the course of MS varies greatly, with some individuals going into spontaneous clinical remission for decades. Others may have few changes on sequential MRIs and either no clinical concomitants or minor sensory changes. Should such individuals, especially those with a clinically isolated syndrome, be advised to start long-term immune-modulating therapy with drugs that do not cure yet can significantly modulate the disease? The question is a difficult one, and there are data indicating that early treatment of such individuals delays the time to development of clinically definite MS.[13,18,19] My approach is to advise treatment in individuals with residua from their first attack; those with evidence of more tissue-destructive processes on their MRIs, such as the presence of "black holes" and atrophy (see Chapter 4); and those with a preponderance of posterior fossa and spinal cord abnormalities. If a person presents with a mild clinically isolated syndrome with full recovery, few if any "black holes" on MRI, and no accumulation of new lesions over time, as documented by serial MRIs, I may delay initiating treatment until a better sense of that person's course of disease is manifest. Such decisions are highly individualized and will also depend on that individual's willingness to wait.

Pregnancy, Breastfeeding, and Disease-Modifying Therapies

Beta-interferons can cause abortions and are Class C drugs according to the FDA. This means they should not be administered to women during pregnancy and should be discontinued prior to attempting to become pregnant. Glatiramer acetate is a Class B drug, meaning that animal studies have not shown adverse effects during pregnancy but no human first-trimester safety data are available. My advice to women wanting to become pregnant is to stop either drug for one or two menstrual cycles prior to initiating pregnancy attempts. The safety of administering beta-interferons or glatiramer acetate during breastfeeding is more uncertain, with no clinical trial data supporting either its safety or its danger. My advise is to avoid either drug during breastfeeding, but to stop breastfeeding and restart disease-modifying therapy if new disease activity is noted either clinically or on MRI.

Beta-Interferons

Interferons are cytokines induced normally in response to inflammation and infection, usually viral infections. There are many types of interferons: alpha, beta, gamma, and tau. The only ones approved for treatment of MS are the human beta-interferons. As noted above, they are one of the mainstays of therapy for relapsing-remitting MS and have been shown to reduce the frequency of relapses and the accumulation of new lesions on MRI.[20–22] Two forms of beta-interferons are available in the United States, beta-interferon 1a and beta-interferon 1b. The differences result from the cells in which the cytokines are produced. Beta-interferon 1a is produced in mammalian cells and is fully glycosylated. Beta-interferon 1b is produced in bacteria, has an amino acid substitution from the normal human beta-interferon, and is not glycosylated. Efficacies of the two forms of beta-interferon at high doses appear to be equivalent. There are differences in efficacy between high-dose and low-dose beta-interferons,[23] as well as differences in the frequency of neutralizing antibodies to beta-interferon (discussed below).

Skin reactions occur with both forms of the subcutaneously injected beta-interferons, consisting mainly of redness, itching, and swelling. These usually subside within hours to days. In some individuals abscesses, either sterile or infected, occur at injections sites. Retraining in injection techniques and skin preparation can minimize such occurrences.

The occurrence of flu-like symptoms is almost universal in patients initiating treatment with beta-interferons. While gradual escalation of dosages and administration of over-the-counter medications can ameliorate such symptoms, they nevertheless can pose a significant side effect to these drugs. Worsening of signs and symptoms of MS can occur during this initial phase of drug administration and patients should be reassured that such worsening most likely is not the result of increasing CNS inflammation.

Neutralizing Antibodies to Beta-Interferon

As with all injectable medications, some individuals will make antibodies to them. At present there are no markers available to detect this genetic diathesis or to predict who will have such a pattern of response. Injection of the beta-interferons elicits antibody responses in many individuals.[24-27] The frequency of such responses varies greatly, depending on how soon after initiation of treatment the testing is done, on the sensitivity of the assay, and on the preparation of beta-interferon being injected. Intramuscular beta-interferon elicits much lower antibody responses than does subcutaneously injected drug, and beta-interferon 1a elicits fewer antibody responses than beta-interferon 1b. Nevertheless, in a recent clinical trial (REGARD trial), persistent levels of antibodies were seen in more than 25% of individuals receiving subcutaneous beta-interferon 1a. Antibodies usually appear after 1 to 2 years on therapy, and in most persons they will persist. If neutralizing antibodies to beta-interferon are not detected after 2 to 3 years on treatment, there is little likelihood they will appear thereafter.

The impact of neutralizing antibodies to beta-interferon on the course of MS remains controversial. However, most MS neurologists agree that having persistently high titers of such antibodies significantly decreases the effectiveness of the drug, in some cases to the level of placebo.[24-27] Persons with persistently high levels of such antibodies should be offered other disease-modifying therapies, such as glatiramer acetate.

This issue is complicated by three factors: in some individuals antibody levels decline over time; persons may develop binding antibodies to beta-interferon but not neutralizing antibodies; and the effects of neutralizing antibodies to beta-interferon may be delayed, so that testing for antibodies is often not initiated until the adverse consequences of such antibodies are apparent. In addition, there is no consensus as to what level of anti-body is sufficient to affect drug efficacy. In some countries where disease-modifying therapies are provided by government-funded health insurance, patients on beta-interferons are tested prospectively 1 and 2 years after starting treatment. If persistent titers of neutralizing antibodies to beta-interferon are noted, patients are switched to another disease-modifying therapy, even though they may be clinically stable. My approach is not to test patients prospectively for the presence of neutralizing antibodies due to the costs of testing and the lack of insurance coverage for such tests. Rather, I follow patients on the beta-interferons carefully, both clinically and with sequential MRIs, and at the first indication of a change in their pattern of response, I test for antibodies. Since antibodies can be transient, I do not test until after at least 1 year of treatment. A second assay may be needed in 6 months to establish antibody persistence. However, if initial levels of antibody are high, persistence is almost always the case, and I will switch to a non-interferon therapy at that time, usually glatiramer acetate.

Table 8.1 summarizes the currently available beta-interferons.

Table 8.1 The Beta-Interferons

Drug	Route	Dosage	Common Side Effects and Treatment
Beta-interferon 1a	IM	30 µg per week	• Flu-like symptoms of muscle aches, headache, fatigue, and fevers are common. Pretreatment with ibuprofen, acetaminophen, or naproxen will help. Symptoms usually subside with time.
			• Low white counts, thrombocytopenia, and thyroid abnormalities can occur. Complete blood counts and liver and thyroid function tests should be obtained every 3 months after starting treatment, with dosage adjustment as needed. If stable at the end of 1 year, testing can be done twice yearly.
			• If after a year there is unexpected worsening in clinical or MRI findings, consider testing for neutralizing antibodies to beta-interferon.
			• Avoid use of this drug during pregnancy. Discontinue use before attempting to become pregnant.
Beta-interferon 1a	Sub-q	22 µg or 44 µg 3 times/ week	• Initial flu-like symptoms are mitigated by starting treatment at a dosage of 11 µg, and escalating weekly by 11 µg per dose until full dosage is achieved. Some patients may tolerate only a 22-µg dose, and prefilled syringes of that dose are available.
			• Low white counts, thrombocytopenia, and thyroid abnormalities can occur. Complete blood counts and liver and thyroid function tests should be obtained every 3 months after starting treatment, with dosage adjustment as needed. If stable at the end of 1 year, testing can be done twice yearly.
			• If after a year there is unexpected worsening in clinical or MRI findings, consider testing for neutralizing antibodies to beta-interferon.
			• Avoid use of this drug during pregnancy. Discontinue use before attempting to become pregnant.
			• Injection site reactions are common, with redness, swelling, and induration. Reactions usually subside over several days and are reduced by injecting the drug at room temperature, pretreating the injection site with warm compresses, and using sites with adequate subcutaneous tissues (see Chapter 6).
Beta-interferon 1b	Sub-q	0.25 mg every other day	• Initial dose is 0.0625 mg for 2 weeks, then the dose is doubled every 2 weeks until full dosage is achieved.
			• Flu-like symptoms of muscle aches, headache, fatigue, and fevers are common. Pretreatment with ibuprofen, acetaminophen, or naproxen will help. Symptoms usually subside with time.

Table 8.1 (Contd.)			
Drug	**Route**	**Dosage**	**Common Side Effects and Treatment**
			• Low white counts, thrombocytopenia, and thyroid abnormalities can occur. Complete blood counts and liver and thyroid function tests should be obtained every 3 months after starting treatment, with dosage adjustment as needed. If stable at the end of 1 year, testing can be done twice yearly.
			• If after a year there is unexpected worsening in clinical or MRI findings, consider testing for neutralizing antibodies to beta-interferon.
			• Avoid use of this drug during pregnancy. Discontinue use before attempting to become pregnant.
			• Injection site reactions are common, with redness, swelling, and induration. Reactions usually subside over several days and are reduced by injecting the drug at room temperature, pretreating the injection site with warm compresses, and using sites with adequate subcutaneous tissues (see Chapter 6).

Glatiramer Acetate

Glatiramer acetate was invented in the 1970s with the intent of inducing an MS-like illness in rodents. It consists of random polymers of four amino acids (alanine, glutamic acid, lysine, and tyrosine) found in high concentrations in a major myelin protein, myelin basic protein. Rather than inducing an MS-like illness, the compound, initially called copolymer I, or Cop I, protected animals from autoimmune CNS disease. The pivotal efficacy trial in humans was conducted in 1995, and thereafter the drug was called glatiramer acetate.[28]

The exact mechanisms of action of the disease-modifying therapies are not known. However, it is probably safe to say that the mechanisms of action of glatiramer acetate are different from those of the beta-interferons. While recent head-to-head trials (REGARD, BEYOND, and BECOME trials) showed equivalent efficacy in terms of clinical and MRI outcomes in groups of MS patients, responses of an individual's disease to the two classes of drugs vary greatly. The new trial data allow one to tell patients about to start treatment that their chances of having a good response to either glatiramer acetate or a high-dose beta-interferon are the same. However, in the absence of biologic markers it is not possible to advise *a priori* which disease-modifying therapy would be best for that person. Since mechanisms of action of the beta-interferons and glatiramer acetate are probably different, an inadequate response to one drug does not preclude an excellent response to the other. Issues in switching disease-modifying therapies will be discussed later in this chapter.

Issues With Glatiramer Acetate

Glatiramer acetate is, in general, well tolerated. There are no flu-like symptoms, nor is there a need to monitor blood counts or liver or thyroid function. All patients on glatiramer acetate make antibodies to the drug, but there are no persuasive data at this time that they affect drug function. The two main difficulties patients have with glatiramer acetate are injection site reactions and the much less common "systemic reaction."

Injection site reactions can be divided into two types, acute reactions and delayed or chronic reactions. The intensity of these reactions and their frequencies vary considerably among individuals. Acute reactions consist of redness, itching, swelling, and induration, which can last for hours to days. Rarely persons develop infections or abscesses[29] (see Chapter 6). The chronic reactions consist of the gradual appearance of injection site subcutaneous induration, over months to years, with loss of subcutaneous fat (lipoatrophy).[30] The result is hard, tough, indented skin that may be very difficult to inject. Acute skin reactions may be eased by pretreating injection sites with warm compresses and injecting the drug at room or body temperature, injecting slowly rather than with an automatic injector, and ensuring that the injection site has sufficient subcutaneous tissue. Inadvertent injection of glatiramer acetate into muscle is extremely painful and can result in large ecchymosis. Little can be done to avoid the chronic skin changes of prolonged glatiramer acetate injection, but using the full expanse of potential injection sites, rather than clustering injections into small areas, may help.

Systemic reactions occur within seconds of drug injections and are characterized by flushing, tachycardia, chest tightness, and shortness of breath. Some individuals also have severe shivering and coldness. Symptoms usually subside within minutes to an hour, no treatment is needed, and there are no serious sequelae. The cause of this reaction is not known, but it is not an allergic reaction and often never recurs. Because many patients note bleeding at the injection site following a systemic reaction, the reaction may result from an inadvertent IV injection of drug. If a person does have a diathesis for systemic reactions, pretreating injection sites with ice to cause vasoconstriction may mitigate this phenomenon.

Table 8.2 summarizes the use of glatiramer acetate.

Second-Line Disease-Modifying Therapies

There are two drugs currently approved in the United States as second-line disease-modifying therapies for MS: the type II topoisomerase inhibitor mitoxantrone and the monoclonal antibody natalizumab. Both are administered IV, and both have unique indications for use and unique side effects.

Mitoxantrone

Mitoxantrone is a type II topoisomerase inhibitor, preventing DNA synthesis and repair. It has been used for decades as treatment for multiple malignancies, in particular metastatic breast cancer, leukemia, and

Table 8.2 Glatiramer Acetate

Route	Dosage	Side Effects and Treatment
Sub-q	20 mg/day	• Acute injection site reactions such as redness, swelling, itching, and induration. Can last for hours to days and vary from person to person and among injection sites too. Treat by injecting the drug at room or body temperature, pretreating injections sites with warm compresses, injecting by hand rather than with an automatic injector, using sites with sufficient subcutaneous tissues, and not injecting into muscle, which is very painful.
		• Chronic skin reactions consist of diffuse induration of the skin with loss of subcutaneous tissue (lipoatrophy). If severe, injections are very difficult. Preventive treatment is best. Distribute injections into the widest possible areas and avoiding narrow clustering of shots. Little can be done once chronic skin changes have occurred.
		• Systemic reactions are uncommon but disquieting. Within seconds of the injection the patient feels hot, flushed, and short of breath, with chest tightness and a rapid heartbeat. In some persons this is followed by severe shivering. Symptoms subside in minutes to an hour, without significant sequelae. This is not an allergic reaction and patients can continue to administer the drug. Avoidance of particular injection sites associated with such reactions may help, as may pretreatment of injection sites with ice or cold compresses to induce vasoconstriction.

non-Hodgkin's lymphoma. It was first used as a treatment for MS in the early 1990s, with the pivotal trial of the drug published in 2002.[4] Mitoxantrone has a profound effect on all proliferating cells and is an immunosuppressant rather than an immune-modulating agent, and thus different from the beta-interferons and glatiramer acetate. Mitoxantrone has a major effect on acute CNS inflammation, reducing the number of contrast-enhancing lesions and the number of relapses. It is approved in the United States for the treatment of rapidly progressive relapsing-remitting MS and for secondary-progressive MS, especially in patients making the transition from relapsing-remitting MS to secondary-progressive MS, and those with rapidly progressive secondary-progressive MS. Because its main actions are anti-inflammatory, mitoxantrone has little effect in the majority of individuals with secondary-progressive MS whose course is gradually progressive over years to decades, with few if any new T2/FLAIR or contrast-enhancing lesions on MRI (see Chapter 3).

Multiple regimens for mitoxantrone administration are described, but the one approved in the United States consists of an IV injection of the drug every 3 months at a dosage of 12 mg/m^2. Because severe dosage-related cardiac toxicity can occur with mitoxantrone,[6,7] the maximum lifetime accumulated dose of drug is 140 mg/m^2, which is usually achieved in 8 to 12 doses. In addition, the drug should not be used in persons with heart disease or cardiac ejection fractions of less than 50%. To avoid cardiac toxicity, the FDA recommends that cardiac ejection fractions be monitored before each dose of drug and that the drug be stopped if there is more than a 10% decrease in the ejection fraction or the ejection fraction falls below 50%.

Since mitoxantrone is a powerful immune suppressant, there is a major decrease in white blood cells several weeks after administration of this drug, greatly increasing the risk of infection. If at all possible I avoid use of colony-stimulating factors such as filgrastim and sargramostim in asymptomatic neutropenic individuals because of the increased risk of inducing an MS relapse.[31] In contrast, patients who develop fevers or other signs of infection while immunosuppressed are immediately evaluated and treated as necessary.

As noted above, dose-related cardiac toxicity, with the appearance of an irreversible cardiomyopathy, is a major risk with this drug. Ejection fraction monitoring should be done before each dose of drug, and the dosage should be reduced or the drug stopped, depending on the results.

A serious risk in persons receiving mitoxantrone is the development of acute and chronic promyelocytic leukemia.[6] The published frequency of this risk is 0.25%, with a usually fatal course.

While low, the risks of mitoxantrone must be carefully weighed against potential benefits.

Natalizumab

Natalizumab is a humanized monoclonal antibody that binds to the cell adherence molecule alpha-4 beta-1 integrin. In so binding it is believed to interfere with the entry of immune cells into the CNS, thus reducing inflammation. Natalizumab has been shown in two clinical trials to have a significant effect on the course of MS, reducing both relapses and the accumulation of disability, and decreasing the appearance of new lesions on MRI.[32,33] It was initially approved for use as a first-line drug for relapsing-remitting MS in November 2004 but was taken off the market in February 2005 due to the appearance of progressive multifocal leukoencephalopathy (PML) in two MS patients also receiving intramuscular beta-interferon 1a. Natalizumab was reapproved by the FDA in March 2006 for use only as monotherapy in persons with relapsing-remitting MS, but with restricted access: all patients have to be enrolled in a risk assessment program called TOUCH in the USA and TIGRIS elsewhere, which are administered by the drug's manufacturer. Because of the risks associated with use of this drug, the FDA suggested it be used primarily in persons with relapsing-remitting MS who do not respond adequately or cannot tolerate treatment with the more usual disease-modifying therapies. Unfortunately, data in support of the effectiveness of natalizumab in this patient population are not available at this time.

In general, patients tolerate infusions of natalizumab well. However, acute infusion reactions have occurred, including anaphylaxis. Chronic or delayed reactions also have been reported, including serum sickness.[10] Approximately 6% of patients on natalizumab develop persistent neutralizing antibodies to the drug, completely abrogating the effectiveness of this agent.[8] These patients also have a higher incidence of infusion reactions. An increased frequency of relapses was noted in patients receiving natalizumab for a short duration, stopping the drug, and then reinstituting it.[34] Liver toxicity, even after only one or two doses of natalizumab, has recently been reported, so careful monitoring of liver function is indicated.

The most serious complications reported with natalizumab treatment are PML and melanoma.[9,11,12] PML occurred in two persons with MS treated with natalizumab while they were participants in a phase III trial of the drug in combination with the intramuscular form of beta-interferon 1a, and recently in two more patients, both on monotherapy with natalizumab for 14 and 17 months respectively. Because the initial two cases occurred in combination with another immune-modulating therapy, current recommendations are to use natalizumab alone. These recommendations will most likely be modified. Prior to the recent report of the two additional cases of PML, the risk of getting PML was estimated at one in 1,000 after at least 18 months of therapy. The difficulty with diagnosing PML in persons with MS is that there are no distinctive changes on MRI or clinically that allow ready differentiation of PML from MS-related disease progression. Identification of the pathogenic Jakob-Creutzfeldt (JC) virus in spinal fluid and/or brain biopsy is needed for definitive diagnosis.

Three cases of malignant melanoma have been reported with the use of natalizumab.[12] One patient was in a phase III trial of the drug and two more were being treated in the community. The two community cases developed melanoma after only short treatment with the drug. Current recommendations are to avoid the use of natalizumab in persons with a history of malignant melanoma or those at high risk for developing this cancer.

Table 8.3 summarizes the second-line immune-modulating therapies.

Switching Disease-Modifying Therapies, or Defining the Insufficient Responder

In a disease as heterogeneous as MS, no one disease-modifying therapy will be effective in all individuals. The fundamental issue is what constitutes "effective." Since none of the current disease-modifying therapies can stop disease progression entirely, at what point should a physician decide to change medications? There are no generally accepted guidelines, and the diversity of opinion is great, even among "experts" in MS. What is generally accepted is that, if at all possible, several criteria should be used: the clinical course of the individual, the findings on the neurologic examination, and the changes on MRI.[35]

The clinical course of MS varies greatly, at times presenting with an "explosive" course, with multiple relapses in a short time. In other patients, attacks occur every several years or even decades. Changes in the course of disease occur even in the absence of treatment, further complicating the issue. However, if a person starts disease-modifying therapy and after a period of at least 9 to 12 months continues to have a pattern of relapses similar to that noted before initiating therapy, with similar frequencies and severities, consideration should be given to switching disease-modifying therapy. Symptoms also are of major importance, with increasing cognitive difficulties, increasing fatigue, and increasing bowel and bladder difficulties

Table 8.3 Second-Line Immune-Modulating Therapies

Drug	Dosage	Protocol	Potential Side Effects
Mitoxantrone	12 mg/m² per dose; lifetime maximum 140 mg/m²	Given IV every 3 months by a chemotherapy-qualified individual, along with 1,000 mg IV methylprednisolone	• Nausea, vomiting, and malaise can occur. These side effects are considerably reduced by administering high-dose IV steroids with the drug. • Neutropenia with risk of infection. During the high-risk periods (1 to 2 weeks after infusion), patients should avoid individuals with infection. Treat fevers or other signs of sepsis immediately, but avoid use of colony-stimulating factors in asymptomatic, neutropenic individuals. • Congestive heart failure. The drug should not be used in persons with cardiac disease. Measure cardiac ejection fractions before starting treatment and then just before each dose. Do not give the drug if the EF is <50% or there is a decline in EF of >10%. • Acute and chronic leukemias. Monitor carefully for signs of blood dyscrasias both before and after treatment is completed.
Natalizumab	300 mg per dose	IV every 4 weeks without any other immune-modulating or immunosuppressive therapies	• Acute sensitivity reactions, such as shortness of breath, tachycardia, flushing, hives, and possibly anaphylaxis. Careful monitoring must be done during each infusion. Drugs and equipment must be readily available to treat hypersensitivity and anaphylactic reactions. • Neutralizing antibodies. More common in persons with acute sensitivity reactions during drug infusions. Test for neutralizing antibodies. If present, stop treatment with the drug. • Malignant melanoma. Do not administer the drug to persons with a history of this cancer or to persons at high risk for developing melanoma. • Progressive multifocal leukoencephalopathy (PML). Administer natalizumab only as monotherapy. Since this infection can manifest years after initiation of treatment, careful clinical monitoring for new or growing MRI lesions or changes in clinical course atypical for MS is needed. CSF examination may also be indicated in patients in whom PML is suspected, with fluid tested for the presence of the pathogenic JC virus. If PML is confirmed, immune reconstitution should be immediately instituted, with removal of any residual natalizumab by multiple plasmaphereses.

all suggesting insufficient responses to medication. As noted above, signs and symptoms of MS may initially increase after starting treatment with one of the beta-interferons, usually in association with the appearance of fatigue, myalgias, and headaches caused by these drugs. Such worsening often improves with time, weeks to months, and need not indicate an insufficient response to therapy.

Changes on the neurologic examination can be found without associated symptoms. Thus, if new findings, such as internuclear ophthalmoplegias, nystagmus, dysmetria, ataxia, or Babinski responses, are noted after 9 to 12 months of disease-modifying therapy and are noted in the absence of fever or other bodily stresses, an insufficient response to medication should be considered.

Changes on MRI may be difficult to determine unless careful attention is given to variation and differences in technique and head placement (see Chapter 4). MRI changes, however, are of great importance. Since all of the disease-modifying therapies reduce the number of new T2/FLAIR lesions as well as the number of lesions showing contrast enhancement, the continued presence of such lesions after 9 to 12 months of therapy is of concern and could indicate an insufficient response to medication. Such changes would be of even greater importance if accompanied by increasing numbers of T1 hypointensities ("black holes") or increasing atrophy, changes shown to be well correlated with increasing disability (see Chapter 4).

If a change in disease-modifying therapy is to be considered, the next question would be, which one? In persons on glatiramer acetate, switching to one of the beta-interferons would be the first choice. In persons on one of the beta-interferons, switching to glatiramer acetate would be the best choice. Several studies have supported such an approach, indicating that patients with an insufficient response to one disease-modifying therapy can be excellent responders to another medication with a different mechanism of action.

What if a person does not respond well to either one of the beta-interferons or glatiramer acetate? Combination therapies have been suggested, but their value in changing the disease course is not fully established at this time.[36] Indeed, some combinations could even increase disease activity (e.g., the combination of high-dose beta-interferons with high-dose statins).[37] Thus, the use of combination therapies should be considered relatively experimental, and referral to an MS center is suggested.

When Should Long-Term Immune-Modulating Therapy Be Stopped?

As described in Chapter 3, most patients with relapsing-remitting MS will gradually have a change in their pattern of disease from one resulting from acute bursts of inflammation to one characterized by a gradual, insidious progression of disability, with low-grade, indolent CNS inflammation, an absence of contrast enhancement on MRI, and a progressive degenerative process with increasing brain atrophy. All of the disease-modifying therapies noted in this chapter, including mitoxantrone, have shown efficacy only in persons with acute inflammation, not in persons with gradually evolving secondary-progressive MS. Therefore, should treatment with disease-modifying therapy be stopped in persons with indolent secondary-progressive MS, and if so when?

This conundrum has faced many physicians providing long-term care to persons with MS, and there is no standard answer. If the reason for stopping treatment was based purely on biologic grounds, the answer would be to stop treatment in anyone who has not had relapses for at least the past 10 years, who has had slow, indolent disease progression, and in whom serial MRIs have not shown new T2/FLAIR lesions or new areas of contrast enhancement. The decision to stop treatment is also easier if an individual has many side effects from the drug or can no longer afford to pay for it. The difficulty is with an individual for whom disease-modifying therapy provides strong emotional support and a feeling of "doing something" when faced with a progressive, incurable illness. In such an individual, stopping therapy can result in feelings of depression and hopelessness and decreasing functional capabilities. While treatment with psychotropic medications is an option, continuing long-term immune-modulating therapy can also be considered.

Future Therapies

While the number of persons with MS, relative to the number with cancer, Alzheimer's disease, stroke, and headache, is small, great efforts are being made by multiple pharmaceutical companies to develop new MS therapies. Almost all efforts are directed at developing drugs that will decrease the acute inflammatory activity present early in the course of the disease. Unfortunately, little effort is being made to develop drugs aimed at treatment of the secondary-progressive phase of the illness. There are multiple reasons for this, including uncertainty about the nature of the pathologic processes present in secondary-progressive MS. However, a major deterrent is the financial cost of conducting clinical trials in this population, there are no immediate MRI markers of efficacy, and long (4 to 5 years) trials may be needed, since the more usual 2- to 3-year trials may be insufficient in this population to show benefit.

Since all of the first-line therapeutic agents for MS are injectables, much effort is being expended to develop oral agents. All are aimed at modulating acute CNS inflammation, although, as noted in Chapter 2, controlling acute inflammation may reduce secondary degenerative mechanisms too. Any acceptable oral medication will need to be at least as effective as the current first-line drugs, as well tolerated, and as safe. Since issues of safety may take years and even decades of use to appraise fully, it is unlikely that any oral drug will immediately displace the current injectable first-line agents. Indeed, two individuals with MS on the drug fingolimod (FTY 720) experienced severe infections and one died.

A similar major effort is being made to develop monoclonal antibodies as MS therapies. As noted above, natalizumab is already an approved agent, and other monoclonals, such as alemtuzumab, rituximab, and daclizumab, are being tested. Such agents have the benefit of infrequent injections (monthly or yearly); they have profound, prolonged actions and they ameliorate disease activity. Unfortunately, all have shown expected and unexpected side effects, some resulting in fatalities (such as a person treated with alemtuzumab who died following an intracranial bleed due to idiopathic thrombocytopenic purpura). Again, issues of long-term safety, tolerance, and assessment of risk:benefit ratios will be important in determining the role of monoclonal antibodies in the long-term management of persons with MS.

References

1. Jacobs L, O'Malley J, Freeman A, Ekes R. Intrathecal interferon reduces exacerbations of multiple sclerosis. *Science*. 1981;214:1026–1028.

2. Interferon beta-1b is effective in relapsing-remitting multiple sclerosis. I. Clinical results of a multicenter, randomized, double-blind, placebo-controlled trial. The IFNB Multiple Sclerosis Study Group. *Neurology*. 1993;43:655–661.

3. Paty DW, Li DK. Interferon beta-1b is effective in relapsing-remitting multiple sclerosis. II. MRI analysis results of a multicenter, randomized, double-blind, placebo-controlled trial. UBC MS/MRI Study Group and the IFNB Multiple Sclerosis Study Group. *Neurology*. 1993;43:662–667.

4. Hartung HP, Gonsette R, Konig N, et al. Mitoxantrone in progressive multiple sclerosis: a placebo-controlled, double-blind, randomised, multicentre trial. *Lancet*. 2002;360:2018–2025.

5. Tremlett HL, Oger J. Ten years of adverse drug reaction reports for the multiple sclerosis immunomodulatory therapies: a Canadian perspective. *Mult Scler*. 2008;14:94–105.

6. Leukaemia due to mitoxantrone. *Prescrire Int*. 2007;16:153–156.

7. Cohen BA, Mikol DD. Mitoxantrone treatment of multiple sclerosis: safety considerations. *Neurology*. 2004;63:S28–32.

8. Calabresi PA, Giovannoni G, Confavreux C, et al. The incidence and significance of anti-natalizumab antibodies: results from AFFIRM and SENTINEL. *Neurology*. 2007;69:1391–1403.

9. Kleinschmidt-DeMasters BK, Tyler KL. Progressive multifocal leukoencephalopathy complicating treatment with natalizumab and interferon beta-1a for multiple sclerosis. *N Engl J Med*. 2005;353:369–374.

10. Krumbholz M, Pellkofer H, Gold R, et al. Delayed allergic reaction to natalizumab associated with early formation of neutralizing antibodies. *Arch Neurol*. 2007;64:1331–1333.

11. Langer-Gould A, Atlas SW, Green AJ, et al. Progressive multifocal leukoencephalopathy in a patient treated with natalizumab. *N Engl J Med*. 2005;353:375–381.

12. Mullen JT, Vartanian TK, Atkins MB. Melanoma complicating treatment with natalizumab for multiple sclerosis. *N Engl J Med*. 2008;358:647–648.

13. Kappos L, Polman CH, Freedman MS, et al. Treatment with interferon beta-1b delays conversion to clinically definite and McDonald MS in patients with clinically isolated syndromes. *Neurology*. 2006;67:1242–1249.

14. Miller D, Barkhof F, Montalban X, et al. Clinically isolated syndromes suggestive of multiple sclerosis, part I: natural history, pathogenesis, diagnosis, and prognosis. *Lancet Neurol*. 2005;4:281–288.

15. Miller D, Barkhof F, Montalban X, et al. Clinically isolated syndromes suggestive of multiple sclerosis, part 2: non-conventional MRI, recovery processes, and management. *Lancet Neurol.* 2005;4:341–348.

16. Sastre-Garriga J, Tintore M, Rovira A, et al. Conversion to multiple sclerosis after a clinically isolated syndrome of the brainstem: cranial magnetic resonance imaging, cerebrospinal fluid and neurophysiological findings. *Mult Scler.* 2003;9:39–43.

17. Siva A. The spectrum of multiple sclerosis and treatment decisions. *Clin Neurol Neurosurg.* 2006;108:333–338.

18. Tintore M. Rationale for early intervention with immunomodulatory treatments. *J Neurol.* 2008;255(Suppl 1):37–43.

19. Frohman EM, Havrdova E, Lublin F, et al. Most patients with multiple sclerosis or a clinically isolated demyelinating syndrome should be treated at the time of diagnosis. *Arch Neurol.* 2006;63:614–619.

20. Jacobs LD, Cookfair DL, Rudick RA, et al. A phase III trial of intramuscular recombinant interferon beta as treatment for exacerbating-remitting multiple sclerosis: design and conduct of study and baseline characteristics of patients. Multiple Sclerosis Collaborative Research Group (MSCRG). *Mult Scler.* 1995;1:118–135.

21. Interferon beta-1b in the treatment of multiple sclerosis: final outcome of the randomized controlled trial. The IFNB Multiple Sclerosis Study Group and the University of British Columbia MS/MRI Analysis Group. *Neurology.* 1995;45:1277–1285.

22. Randomised double-blind placebo-controlled study of interferon beta-1a in relapsing/remitting multiple sclerosis. PRISMS (Prevention of Relapses and Disability by Interferon beta-1a Subcutaneously in Multiple Sclerosis) Study Group. *Lancet.* 1998;352:1498–1504.

23. Schwid SR, Panitch HS. Full results of the Evidence of Interferon Dose-Response-European North American Comparative Efficacy (EVIDENCE) study: a multicenter, randomized, assessor-blinded comparison of low-dose weekly versus high-dose, high-frequency interferon beta-1a for relapsing multiple sclerosis. *Clin Ther.* 2007;29:2031–2048.

24. Durelli L, Barbero P, Bergui M, et al. MRI activity and neutralising antibody as predictors of response to interferon beta treatment in multiple sclerosis. *J Neurol Neurosurg Psychiatry.* 2008;79:646–651.

25. Hartung HP, Polman C, Bertolotto A, et al. Neutralising antibodies to interferon beta in multiple sclerosis: expert panel report. *J Neurol.* 2007;254:827–837.

26. Malucchi S, Gilli F, Caldano M, et al. Predictive markers for response to interferon therapy in patients with multiple sclerosis. *Neurology.* 2008 March 25;70 (13 pt 2):1119–1127.

27. Sorensen PS, Koch-Henriksen N, Bendtzen K. Are ex vivo neutralising antibodies against IFN-beta always detrimental to therapeutic efficacy in multiple sclerosis? *Mult Scler.* 2007;13:616–621.

28. Johnson KP, Brooks BR, Cohen JA, et al. Copolymer 1 reduces relapse rate and improves disability in relapsing-remitting multiple sclerosis: results of a phase III multicenter, double-blind placebo-controlled trial. The Copolymer 1 Multiple Sclerosis Study Group. *Neurology.* 1995;45:1268–1276.

29. Bosca I, Bosca M, Belenguer A, et al. Necrotising cutaneous lesions as a side effect of glatiramer acetate. *J Neurol.* 2006;253:1370–1371.

30. Edgar CM, Brunet DG, Fenton P, et al. Lipoatrophy in patients with multiple sclerosis on glatiramer acetate. *Can J Neurol Sci.* 2004;31:58–63.

31. Openshaw H, Stuve O, Antel JP, et al. Multiple sclerosis flares associated with recombinant granulocyte colony-stimulating factor. *Neurology.* 2000;54:2147–2150.

32. Miller DH, Soon D, Fernando KT, et al. MRI outcomes in a placebo-controlled trial of natalizumab in relapsing MS. *Neurology.* 2007;68:1390–1401.

33. Polman CH, O'Connor PW, Havrdova E, et al. A randomized, placebo-controlled trial of natalizumab for relapsing multiple sclerosis. *N Engl J Med.* 2006;354:899–910.

34. Vellinga MM, Castelijns JA, Barkhof F, et al. Postwithdrawal rebound increase in T2 lesional activity in natalizumab-treated MS patients. *Neurology.* 2008;70:1150–1151.

35. Freedman MS, Patry DG, Grand'Maison F, et al. Treatment optimization in multiple sclerosis. *Can J Neurol Sci.* 2004;31:157–168.

36. Gold R. Combination therapies in multiple sclerosis. *J Neurol.* 2008;255 (Suppl 1):51–60.

37. Birnbaum G, Cree B, Altafullah I, et al. Combining beta interferon and atorvastatin may increase disease activity in multiple sclerosis. *Neurology.* 2008 June 4 [E-pub before print].

Chapter 9

Management of Multiple Sclerosis Symptoms

Much to many a neurologist's surprise, studies on the treatment of MS symptoms showed that most physicians fail to address this aspect of the disease.[1] While treatment of the underlying pathologic process is of major importance, failure to treat MS symptoms can result in a seriously compromised quality of life for both patients and their families, as well as increased disability.

Symptoms of MS vary considerably among individuals and change over time. Most MS symptoms can be modified, but only a few can be eliminated completely. Severity of symptoms, duration, and ability to tolerate symptom-relieving medications are all important variables.[2–4]

Learning the full spectrum of symptoms in an individual is a challenge, given the constraints on time that often are part of a clinic visit. Symptom diversity and complexity require careful questioning and interpretation, and there is no substitute for time. A useful tool in our practice is to send each patient a questionnaire, detailing different aspects of MS, from cognition, to fatigue, to pain, to spasms, to medication lists and side effects. Questionnaires are mailed back to us prior to the patient's visit and reviewed. This allows individuals to describe their difficulties at their leisure and allows us to focus on areas of greatest concern at the time of their visit. A questionnaire can be completed at the time of the clinic visit, but this may reduce face-to-face time between the patient and health care provider.

While medications clearly can alleviate symptoms, there is no "free lunch" when it comes to side effects from these drugs. All medications have the potential not only for side effects but also for interfering with the effectiveness of other drugs. Often dosages of symptom-managing medications are limiting, requiring compromises or the use of multiple drugs. For some symptoms nondrug approaches are the best and initial approach to management. This is especially true for the symptoms of fatigue and spasticity. Again, asking, listening, and allowing enough time are needed to maximize treatment benefits.

Fatigue

Not all symptoms associated with MS are directly related to CNS inflammation. This is best exemplified by fatigue, one of the most pervasive of

MS symptoms and one of the most complex.[2,3] Fatigue can certainly result from intrinsic CNS inflammation, but other confounding variables such as drug side effects, mood alterations (in particular depression), deconditioning, obesity, lack of restorative sleep (e.g., sleep apnea), metabolic changes such anemia, thyroid dysfunction, and adrenal suppression due to steroids, and chronic infection must be considered.[5–9] Dissecting out these variables is a challenge, and each requires a different treatment.

One of the most effective treatments for fatigue, whether related directly to MS, to deconditioning, to obesity, and to an extent to depression, is regular exercise.[10–14] Persuading persons with fatigue to exercise can be more of a challenge than even dissecting the variables of this symptom. The usual response is, "I'm too tired to exercise," "I'm too busy," "My difficulties with walking, balance, and coordination get worse," "I don't know how," or "I don't have the equipment." The four best responses to these objections are as follows:

1. Do something, no matter how trivial.
2. Keep it as simple as possible, so that exercise becomes as much a part of the daily routine as putting on one's clothes. An example of such a routine would be to stretch upon awakening, address bodily needs then do some form of cardiac and muscle strengthening exercises (free weights, elastic bands, yoga, Pilates, Tai Chi, treadmill, etc.). Activities can be varied, with a cardiac workout one day and a muscle strengthening workout on alternate days.
3. Do things very gradually to avoid the consequences of "overdoing it."
4. Have realistic expectations: exercise is not "magical" but is an important approach to maximizing energy and function.

Obviously, what persons can do will depend on the extent of their disabilities. Fortunately, in the past decade multiple exercise regimens for persons with disabilities have become available, either in book format or on DVDs. Joining an exercise club is acceptable, as is swimming, but from past experience these more complicated approaches are unlikely to be continued over the long term. The emphasis should be on exercise as something to be done regularly, "until age 99," with a goal of 30 minutes (or more) five days per week. The advice of a physical therapist or an exercise physiologist, experienced in the unique aspects of MS care, can be very valuable. Almost always, persons doing regular exercise note improved energy, better mood, and better function.

Depression

As noted in Chapter 6, many persons with MS have mood disturbances, especially depression.[5,15,16] The risk of suicide is many times higher in persons with MS than in the general population, and every person with suspected depression should be asked about the presence of suicidal thoughts and the extent of their implementation.[17–20] If present, immediate referral to a psychiatrist should be considered. The diagnosis of depression and its treatment are described in Chapter 6 and below.

Pain

Pain, like fatigue, can have multifactorial causes in persons with MS.[21,22] Pain can occur as a direct result of inflammation and demyelination in sensory nerves, such as the dorsal roots and trigeminal nerve; in sensory tracts, such as the spinothalamic tracts; and in thalamic nuclei. However, pain also can result from spasticity and from changes in joints and other musculoskeletal structures as a result of weakness (e.g., knee hyperextension), restricted range of motion (e.g., "frozen" shoulders), or altered walking dynamics (e.g., hip and back pain). Pain also can result from comorbidities associated with MS, such as back pain from vertebral body compressive fractures resulting from osteoporosis, or carpal tunnel syndrome as a result of hand contractures. As noted for fatigue, management of pain will depend on the causes of the discomfort.

Spasticity

While spasticity in MS is almost always the result of interruption or dysfunction of the corticospinal pathways, other factors can significantly exacerbate this symptom complex. The most common are infections, especially of the urinary tract,[23] skin breakdown in the lower extremities, and starting disease-modifying therapies, in particular the beta-interferons. Thus, analyses and treatment will differ in different individuals.

Sexual Dysfunction

Difficulties with libido, arousal, and ability to have orgasm can occur in combination with bowel and bladder changes or in isolation and are common in persons with MS.[24–28] For many patients and health care providers, talking about such issues is difficult. For meaningful treatment of sexual difficulties, such reluctance should be overcome. Discussion of issues with the sexual partner and agreement on suggested methods of treatment also are essential for treatment success.

Loss of libido is common, and multiple factors can produce this. Some important ones are depression, with loss of self-esteem and perceived sexual attractiveness; fatigue; fear of having difficulty with arousal; side effects of medications, especially SSRIs; and physical impairments preventing sexual activity. Difficulties with arousal usually result from impaired perineal or penile sensation. In women, this results in impaired lubrication, pain with intercourse, and difficulties with orgasm. In men, erectile dysfunction and difficulty achieving orgasm are common.[26] Treatment of these symptoms is described below.

With increased sexual activity comes an increased risk of UTIs. Management of this risk involves education regarding the need for perineal washing before intercourse, voiding before and after intercourse, and avoiding prolonged, overly vigorous intercourse. Some women lose bladder control at the moment of orgasm. Bladder emptying and use of anticholinergic medications prior to having sexual relations can be of benefit.

Conclusion

Table 9.1 reviews some of the most common and important symptoms directly related to the CNS inflammation of MS and approaches to their management.

Treating the many symptoms of MS is as difficult a challenge as modifying the course disease. Paying careful attention to details and allowing sufficient time for patient–physician interaction remain the foundation for success in this area.

Table 9.1 Symptom Management in MS

Symptom	Treatment	Potential Difficulties
Fatigue	1. The first goal is to correct any metabolic abnormalities, such as anemia, thyroid dysfunction, adrenal hypofunction, and chronic infections, such as sinusitis, gingivitis, and cystitis.	1. Adjusting hormonal status and determining adequate control of recurrent infections can be difficult.
	2. Addressing disorders of mood, especially depression and anxiety, with appropriate counseling and medications (such as venlafaxine and citalopram)	2. Reluctance of the patient to acknowledge that there is an issue with mood and that it should be treated; worsening depression after treatment
	3. Addressing disorders of sleep, such as nocturnal myoclonus, "restless legs," spasms, obstructive sleep apnea, early morning awakening, and nocturia (see Chapter 6)	3. Potential side effects of medications, inability to use breathing devices for persons with obstructive sleep apnea, and anticipation of side effects as can occur with restless legs syndrome
	4. Gradually progressive exercises, both aerobic and resistive, with a goal of a half-hour five times per week	4. Too rapid an escalation of exercises may result in worsening MS symptoms and more fatigue. Doing incorrect exercises may cause injury.
	5. If all the above fail, stimulatory medications can be considered. Some antidepressants, such as bupropion and venlafaxine, have this property. Other drugs are amantadine, 100 mg bid, and modafinil, 200 to 300 mg per day.[8,29] In refractory cases use of stimulants such as methylphenidate can be considered.	5. As with all stimulants, insomnia, anxiety, tachycardia, hypertension, and panic attacks are potential side effects. Tolerance to stimulatory medications is common. Changing from one drug to another may help, as can "drug holidays," brief (1 to 2 weeks) periods off a drug, followed by re-institution.

| Table 9.1 *(continued)* |

Symptom	Treatment	Potential Difficulties

Pain	1. For central or neurogenic pain (trigeminal neuralgia, causalgia, hyperesthetic pain, radicular pain):
	
	  a. Antiepileptic drugs (carbamazepine, oxcarbazepine, gabapentin, topiramate, pregabalin), tricyclic antidepressants (amitriptyline, nortriptyline), and duloxetine
	
	  b. As a last resort, long-acting opiates, such as fentanyl and methadone, can be considered.
		1a. Side effects of all medications may be limiting, such as sedation, fatigue, and imbalance. Taking medications with food may decrease the rate of absorption and allow higher dosing.
		
		1b. Tolerance of drugs, in particular opiates, can occur, with progressively higher doses needed to achieve benefits. Very gradual tapering off drugs should be done if switching from one drug to another is required. Drug dependency and abuse of opiates is uncommon in persons with MS but does occur.

	2. For pain due to spasticity and cramping:
	
	  a. Adequate hydration with sufficient intake of calcium (dairy products or calcium tablets, 600 mg bid, taken with food, and vitamin D, 1,000 IU per day), potassium (figs, apricots, all bran, bananas, raisins, tomatoes, sultanas, wheat germ), and magnesium (black beans, raw broccoli, halibut, and cooked spinach)
	
	  b. Stretching of tightened muscles daily, slowly and gently, for at least 30 to 45 seconds each. Training may be necessary.
	
	  c. Medications, such as baclofen (10 to 20 mg per dose, starting low and increasing slowly to 80 to 100 mg/day in divided doses), tizanidine (2 to 8 mg per dose, initially hs, then gradually advance as tolerated to a maximum of 32 mg/day), gabapentin, in gradually increasing dosages to 900 to 1,800 mg per day, benzodiazepines (clonazepam, diazepam, starting with hs dosing and gradually increasing to daytime dosing), cyclobenzaprine (10 mg bid), metaxalone (800 mg tid or qid, on an empty stomach)
		2a. Achieving adequate hydration in persons with bladder difficulties can be hard to achieve, as often such individuals restrict fluid intake to minimize bladder symptoms.
		
		2b. Muscle and joint injury due to inadequate training in muscle stretching and lengthening procedures
		
		2c. Medication side effects can be limiting, especially constipation with calcium, weakness and fatigue with higher doses of baclofen, benzodiazepines, and muscle relaxants, and sedation with tizanidine and benzodiazepines.

Table 9.1 (continued)

Symptom	Treatment	Potential Difficulties
	d. For spasticity refractory to the above measures, careful injection of botulinum toxin into the most affected muscles, such as leg adductor muscles, may be of benefit.	2d. Injection of botulinum toxin into muscles can result in marked muscle weakness, at times extending to muscles beyond the areas of injection. Thus, the least amount of botulinum toxin should be used.
	e. If spasticity is too widespread to be treated with individual muscle treatment, use of an intrathecal baclofen pump can be of great value.	2e. Placement of an intrathecal baclofen pump, while a powerful tool, carries with it the risks of all implanted devices, namely infection, pump failure, catheter kinking and breakage, and the need for dosage monitoring and pump refilling.
	3. Pain due to musculoskeletal discomfort from limb weakness, altered walking dynamics, joint restrictions (e.g, "frozen" shoulders):	
	a. Initially physical therapy is the mainstay of treatment, with emphasis on muscle strengthening and stretching, and instructions in the proper use of assistive devices (canes, walkers).	3a. Delay in initiation of joint contractures can result in permanent disabilities.
	b. Orthotics can be of great help, especially ankle–foot orthoses, knee and ankle braces, modification of cane handles to prevent median and ulnar nerve dysfunction, and shoe orthotics. Weight and flexibility of devices should be tailored to individual needs, with avoidance of large, heavy devices, if possible.	3b. Uncomfortable and poorly adjusted orthotics can reduce mobility and increase disability, and may not be used at all.
	c. Adequate pain and muscle relaxant medications to allow maximal joint mobilization and stretching	3c. Medication side effects of sedation, fatigue, and increasing weakness can be limiting.
Spasticity	Similar to the descriptions of treatment of pain due to spasticity, noted above	Similar to the descriptions of treatment of pain due to spasticity, noted above
Bladder difficulties	1. Bladder urgency, frequency, loss of control, and incomplete emptying are common MS symptoms.	
	a. Initial, drug-free approaches to treatment would be timed voiding—that is, voiding by the clock rather than waiting until bladder contractions occur.	1a. Recurrent UTIs are common and may result from incomplete bladder emptying resulting from use of anticholinergic medications and in women

Symptom	Treatment	Potential Difficulties
	In women with MS who have had children, there can be a weakening of the pelvic floor musculature, with resulting stress and urge incontinence unrelated to neurologic disease. Training in pelvic floor strengthening exercises and biofeedback by an experienced physical therapist can greatly improve bladder symptoms.	insufficient attention to voiding after sexual intercourse and to proper wiping after bowel movements (front to back is recommended).
	b. While most bladder difficulties in persons with MS are due to spinal cord dysfunction, bladder sensation is often reduced in persons with MS, with loss of the usual symptoms of a UTI. Thus, first test for the presence of a UTI, and treat if present. While chronic bacteriuria is common, bacterial suppressant medications, such as nitrofurantoin and low doses of trimethoprim/sulfamethoxazole, can reduce bacterial load and improve bladder symptoms.	
	c. Next, determine bladder size with a bladder ultrasound. Symptoms alone cannot differentiate a small spastic bladder from a large atonic bladder. Treatments are diametrically different.	
	d. Small, spastic bladders are treated with anticholinergics. Multiple medications are available. The most commonly used drugs are oxybutynin, either in pill form or patches that are changed every 3 to 4 days, toleridine, trospium, solifenacin, and darifenacin. Recent studies in patients refractory to treatment with oral medications suggest that injection of botulinum toxin into detrusor muscles is effective in reducing bladder urgency and frequency, but not in reducing postvoid residuals.[30–32] Such use is "off label" and should be considered experimental at this time.	1d. Multiple side effects can occur with use of anticholinergics. Most common are dry mouth and orthostatic dizziness. Altered cognition is also possible in persons with already compromised cognitive abilities. Constipation also can increase. Proper bowel regimens, as described below, may be needed. Use of larger doses of botulinum toxin to treat detrusor overactivity can result in a flaccid bladder with overflow into rectal muscles, with resulting loss of sphincter control.

Table 9.1 (continued)

Symptom	Treatment	Potential Difficulties
	e. Large, atonic bladders are initially treated with alpha-adrenergic blockers, such as alfuzosin, tamsulosin, and doxazosin. Monitoring with bladder scans may be needed to ensure efficacy. If insufficient emptying is still noted, intermittent self-catheterization or chronic catheterization may be needed.	1e. Use of alpha-adrenergic agents can increase difficulties with bladder urgency and control, and dosages may need to be adjusted or medications changed.
	f. If bladder symptoms are refractory to treatments, urologic evaluation may be needed to determine the presence of other urinary tract abnormalities such as bladder and renal calculi, hydronephrosis due to chronic bladder retention, urethral structures, and in males prostatic hypertrophy.	
Bowel difficulties	Constipation is common in patients with MS.[27,33] Defining constipation is important. Daily bowel movements are not necessarily the goal, but movements at least every 3 days is. Again, causes of constipation are multifactorial. Among the most common, other than spinal cord dysfunction, are insufficient dietary bulk, insufficient dietary liquids, lack of a consistent evacuation regimen, and lack of exercise.	
	a. Lack of dietary bulk is easily addressed with use of psyllium or other bulk agents, or a change in diet to one with more high-fiber foods, such as apples, vegetables, and salads.	1a. Food high in fiber can cause bloating in some individuals and diarrhea in others. The latter is especially unpleasant, given already existing issues of urgency and loss of control. Balancing constipation and diarrhea can be a challenge but is possible.
	b. Lack of sufficient liquid intake also is important, but it may be difficult to persuade patients with bladder symptoms to drink more, since many restrict fluid intake to minimize bladder symptoms. However, an achievable goal would be to advise patients to drink enough liquids to maintain urine color in the light yellow range, and to consume more liquids if urine color darkens.	1b. Since bladder and bowel dysfunction are often associated, drugs to used treat bladder dysfunction, such as anticholinergics, can worsen constipation. Again, a balance of benefits versus side effects should be sought.

Symptom	Treatment	Potential Difficulties
	c. Establishing a good bowel regimen involves using the gastrocolic reflex (colonic contractions after gastric filling), regular times for evacuation, and patience. Trying to evacuate at the same time each day, after a meal, helps, and patients should be advised not to suppress bowel urges, as continued suppression may result in loss of this important reflex.	1c. Increasing fluid intake may worsen difficulties in persons with associated bladder difficulties with a reluctance to drink more. Use of stool softeners, such as docusate, allow some reduction in fluid intake while still avoiding stool inspissation.
	d. Exercise as a means of increasing bowel peristalsis is well described, and the approaches to exercise are described above in the section on management of fatigue and in Chapter 6.	
	e. If none of the above approaches is of sufficient benefit, medications can help. Use of a stool softener, such as docusate, is of value. Initial and then occasional use of a mild stimulatory suppository, such as glycerin or bisacodyl, helps to establish an evacuation schedule. Occasional use of enemas can help restore function, especially if stool is very hard. Occasional use of irritative and osmotic agents, such as senna, lactulose, and polyethylene glycol, is effective. However, chronic use should be avoided, as dependence on these agents occurs quickly.	
Sexual difficulties	1. Loss of libido due to depression, loss of self-esteem, and perceived lack of sexual attractiveness are best addressed with counseling and, if needed, antidepressants with a minimum of sexual depressant effects, such as bupropion.	1. Reluctance to discuss sexual issues and reluctance to discuss the results of treatment recommendations are obstacles that may be impossible to overcome. Increased sexual activity is associated with an increased risk of UTIs. Instruction in perineal hygiene, voiding after intercourse, and avoiding prolonged intercourse should be provided. Some women experience uncontrollable bladder emptying with orgasms. Emptying the bladder before intercourse and using anticholinergic drugs may help avoid this.

Table 9.1 (*continued*)		
Symptom	**Treatment**	**Potential Difficulties**
	2. Difficulties with arousal and orgasm due to loss of perineal sensation are treated differently in men and women.	
	a. In woman, use of a vibrator or other device, such as a clitoral suction device, can provide the increased vaginal and clitoral stimulation needed to achieve orgasm. Changing position during sex, with the woman on top, may allow her to better stimulate herself. Use of a water-based lubricant also decreases irritation and discomfort.	
	b. For men, use of drugs enhancing the vasodilating effects of nitric oxide (phosphodiesterase-5 [PDE5] inhibitors) helps with erectile dysfunction. These include oral agents, such as sildenafil, vardenafil, and tadalafil, and penile injection with alprostadil. If side effects of these drugs are not tolerated, penile vacuum devices and penile rings are effective. Finally, penile implants, either semirigid or permanent, can be considered.	2b. Vasodilating drugs used to treat erectile dysfunction may be contraindicated in persons on antihypertensive medications due to the risk of systemic hypotension. Side effects of these vasodilating drugs, such as headache, visual changes, and facial flushing, also may be limiting.
	3. Drug related impairment of sexual function is frequent, especially with SSRIs. Changing drugs or lowering dosages are options.	
	4. Ways to reduce fatigue, spasticity, and bladder symptoms are discussed elsewhere in this chapter.	
Cognitive changes	Changes in cognition are common and take many forms, from difficulties with short-term memory, to inability to concentrate and multitask, to difficulties with executive functions, such as difficulty making decisions or making inappropriate decisions. Causes are multifactorial and can result from changes in mood, such as anxiety, stress, and depression; side effects of medications, such as sedating or anticholinergic drugs; changes	

Symptom	Treatment	Potential Difficulties
	in brain integrity due to neuronal and axonal losses from MS; fatigue with nonrestorative sleep; or a combination of all four.	
	a. Distinguishing between etiologies may be difficult. In such instances, neuropsychometric testing can be of great value, also allowing quantitation of deficits.	1a. Decreasing medications that could impair cognition may result in compromising control of other symptoms. Prioritizing with the patient's assistance is needed, with reduction of doses to acceptable levels.
	b. Changes in mood are treated as noted in previous chapters, with counseling, antidepressants, usually of the SSRI or SSNRI class, or anti-anxiety medications such as lorazepam, alprazolam, or buspirone.	1b. Use of analeptic or CNS stimulatory drugs can increase anxiety reactions, with further impairment of cognition.
	c. Symptom management of fatigue and nonrestorative sleep are described above under management of fatigue.	
	d. Unfortunately, there are no firmly established treatments for changes in cognition due to progressive loss of brain tissue. Use of donepezil, 5 to 10 mg/day, has been described and may be of benefit in some individuals.[34] Liberal use of notes, calendars, and other memory assistive devices, such as electronic organizers, may also help.	
Heat intolerance	As core temperature increases, nonsaltatory conduction along demyelinated nerves decreases and MS symptoms get worse (mainly fatigue and weakness). This can occur in a setting of infection with fevers, after exercising, and with increased ambient temperatures. Elevated ambient temperatures can seriously limit the activities of a person with MS, but the following techniques help:	None of the recommendations may be sufficient to allow prolonged activities in high-temperature environments. Patients should limit activities to cooler times of the day or should limit themselves to only short periods of activity.
	1. Wearing a large, full-brimmed, light-colored hat when in the sun will reflect heat from the brain.	

Table 9.1 *(continued)*

Symptom	Treatment	Potential Difficulties
	2. Wearing loose-fitting, light-colored, heat-reflecting clothing	
	3. Having a cool drink available at all times to reduce core temperature	
	4. Using nonconstrictive cooling devices, such as water-soaked neck bands, neck bands with ice packs, or small electric fans that spray water on face and arms. Cooling vests containing ice packs are available, but most are bulky and constrictive and increase body temperature as they lose their cooling abilities.	4. Some of the more elaborate cooling devices may be too expensive for some individuals, and larger devices such as cooling vests can restrict movement and increase body temperature as they warm up.
	5. Putting bare feet in a tub of cool (not cold) water is remarkably cooling and a rapid way of reducing core temperature.	
Tremors	This symptom complex is especially difficult to manage and can be a source of significant disability. Tremors can involve the arms, legs, and trunk, and medications have limited value in their management. Some that have proved useful in some individuals are:	Slow tapering off all of these medications is necessary to avoid withdrawal symptoms (and potential cardiac difficulties in the case of the beta-blocker propranolol).
	a. Clonazepam, 0.5 mg initially once per day. As tolerance to the sedative effects of the drug is noted, dosages can be increased to bid and tid.	a and b. Sedating side effects from clonazepam and primidone are limiting.
	b. Primidone, 50 mg/day initially. The dosage can be increased to bid and tid as needed or as tolerated.	
	c. Propranolol, 40 mg bid, with gradually increasing dosages, as needed, to a maximum of 320 mg/day	c. Hypotension and bradycardia can be limiting with use of propranolol.
	d. In severe, drug-refractory cases of tremor, thalamotomy and deep brain stimulation have been tried, with some benefit.[35–37]	d. While short-term benefits may accrue from neurosurgical intervention, in a progressive disease such as MS, results over time decrease and residua and complications of surgery may add to disability.

References

1. Vickrey BG, Shatin D, Wolf SM, et al. Management of multiple sclerosis across managed care and fee-for-service systems. *Neurology*. 2000;55:1341–1349.

2. Rayton HJ, Rossman HS. Managing the symptoms of multiple sclerosis: A multi-modal approach. *Clin Ther*. 2006;28:445–460.

3. O'Connor P. Symptom management. *Adv Neurol*. 2006;98:227–255.

4. Schapiro RT. Managing symptoms of multiple sclerosis. *Neurol Clin*. 2005;23:177–187.

5. Beiske AG, Svensson E, Sandanger I, et al. Depression and anxiety amongst multiple sclerosis patients. *Eur J Neurol*. 2008;15:239–245.

6. Chwastiak LA, Gibbons LE, Ehde DM, et al. Fatigue and psychiatric illness in a large community sample of persons with multiple sclerosis. *J Psychosom Res*. 2005;59:291–298.

7. Kaynak H, Altintas A, Kaynak D, et al. Fatigue and sleep disturbance in multiple sclerosis. *Eur J Neurol*. 2006;13:1333–1339.

8. Rosenberg JH, Shafor R. Fatigue in multiple sclerosis: a rational approach to evaluation and treatment. *Curr Neurol Neurosci Rep*. 2005;5:140–146.

9. Stanton BR, Barnes F, Silber E. Sleep and fatigue in multiple sclerosis. *Mult Scler*. 2006;12:481–486.

10. Brown TR, Kraft GH. Exercise and rehabilitation for individuals with multiple sclerosis. *Phys Med Rehabil Clin North Am*. 2005;16:513–555.

11. Gallien P, Nicolas B, Robineau S, et al. Physical training and multiple sclerosis. *Ann Readapt Med Phys*. 2007;50:369–376.

12. McCullagh R, Fitzgerald AP, Murphy RP, Cooke G. Long-term benefits of exercising on quality of life and fatigue in multiple sclerosis patients with mild disability: a pilot study. *Clin Rehabil*. 2008;22:206–214.

13. Petajan JH, Gappmaier E, White AT, et al. Impact of aerobic training on fitness and quality of life in multiple sclerosis. *Ann Neurol*. 1996;39:432–441.

14. White LJ, Dressendorfer RH. Exercise and multiple sclerosis. *Sports Med*. 2004;34:1077–1100.

15. Chwastiak LA, Ehde DM. Psychiatric issues in multiple sclerosis. *Psychiatr Clin North Am*. 2007;30:803–817.

16. Wilken JA, Sullivan C. Recognizing and treating common psychiatric disorders in multiple sclerosis. *Neurologist*. 2007;13:343–354.

17. Feinstein A. An examination of suicidal intent in patients with multiple sclerosis. *Neurology*. 2002;59:674–678.

18. Stenager EN, Koch-Henriksen N, Stenager E. Risk factors for suicide in multiple sclerosis. *Psychother Psychosom*. 1996;65:86–90.

19. Turner AP, Williams RM, Bowen JD, et al. Suicidal ideation in multiple sclerosis. *Arch Phys Med Rehabil*. 2006;87:1073–1078.

20. Wallin MT, Wilken JA, Turner AP, et al. Depression and multiple sclerosis: Review of a lethal combination. *J Rehabil Res Dev*. 2006;43:45–62.

21. O'Connor AB, Schwid SR, Herrmann DN, et al. Pain associated with multiple sclerosis: Systematic review and proposed classification. *Pain*. 2008 July; 137(1):96–111.

22. Ramirez-Lassepas M, Tulloch JW, Quinones MR, Snyder BD. Acute radicular pain as a presenting symptom in multiple sclerosis. *Arch Neurol*. 1992;49:255–258.

23. Edlich RF, Westwater JJ, Lombardi SA, et al. Multiple sclerosis and asymptomatic urinary tract infection. *J Emerg Med.* 1990;8:25–28.

24. Demirkiran M, Sarica Y, Uguz S, et al. Multiple sclerosis patients with and without sexual dysfunction: are there any differences? *Mult Scler.* 2006;12:209–214.

25. Gruenwald I, Vardi Y, Gartman I, et al. Sexual dysfunction in females with multiple sclerosis: quantitative sensory testing. *Mult Scler.* 2007;13:95–105.

26. Landtblom AM. Treatment of erectile dysfunction in multiple sclerosis. *Expert Rev Neurother.* 2006;6:931–935.

27. Nortvedt MW, Riise T, Frugard J, et al. Prevalence of bladder, bowel and sexual problems among multiple sclerosis patients two to five years after diagnosis. *Mult Scler.* 2007;13:106–112.

28. Tzortzis V, Skriapas K, Hadjigeorgiou G, et al. Sexual dysfunction in newly diagnosed multiple sclerosis women. *Mult Scler.* 2008 Jan. 31 [E-pub before print].

29. Zifko UA. Management of fatigue in patients with multiple sclerosis. *Drugs.* 2004;64:1295–1304.

30. Gallien P, Reymann JM, Amarenco G, et al. Placebo-controlled, randomised, double-blind study of the effects of botulinum A toxin on detrusor sphincter dyssynergia in multiple sclerosis patients. *J Neurol Neurosurg Psychiatry.* 2005;76:1670–1676.

31. Game X, Castel-Lacanal E, Bentaleb Y, et al. Botulinum toxin A detrusor injections in patients with neurogenic detrusor overactivity significantly decrease the incidence of symptomatic urinary tract infections. *Eur Urol.* 2008;53:613–618.

32. Kalsi V, Gonzales G, Popat R, et al. Botulinum injections for the treatment of bladder symptoms of multiple sclerosis. *Ann Neurol.* 2007;62:452–457.

33. Bywater A, While A. Management of bowel dysfunction in people with multiple sclerosis. *Br J Commun Nurs.* 2006;11:333–340.

34. Christodoulou C, Melville P, Scherl WF, et al. Effects of donepezil on memory and cognition in multiple sclerosis. *J Neurol Sci.* 2006;245:127–136.

35. Schuurman PR, Bosch DA, Merkus MP, Speelman JD. Long-term follow-up of thalamic stimulation versus thalamotomy for tremor suppression. *Mov Disord.* 2008;23:1146–1153.

36. Koch M, Mostert J, Heersema D, De Keyser J. Tremor in multiple sclerosis. *J Neurol.* 2007;254:133–145.

37. Schuurman PR, Bosch DA, Bossuyt PM, et al. A comparison of continuous thalamic stimulation and thalamotomy for suppression of severe tremor. *N Engl J Med.* 2000;342:461–468.

Further Reading

Koch M, Mostert J, Meersema D, et al. Tremor in multiple sclerosis. *J Neurol.* 2007;254(2):133–145.

Mills RJ, Yap L, Young CA. Treatment for ataxia in multiple sclerosis. *Cochrane Database Syst Rev,* 2007(1): p. CD005029.

Zorzon M, Zivadinov R, Locatelli L, et al. Long-term effects of intravenous high dose methylprednisolone pulses on bone mineral density in patients with multiple sclerosis. *Eur J Neurol.* 2005;12:550–556.

Chapter 10

Complementary Therapies for Multiple Sclerosis

Providing truly comprehensive care to persons with MS requires the services of health professionals other than physicians. There are multiple aspects of disease management that cannot be addressed as part of an individual's visit to the physician's office, and these additional aspects of disease management are the subject of this chapter.

Individual needs will vary greatly depending on the phase of the person's illness (e.g., newly diagnosed, or entering the secondary-progressive phase of their disease), their degree of disability, and the support available from family and friends. Availability of services and financial resources also vary greatly, potentially putting more burden on caregivers and necessitating compromises. In an ideal world, all services described below would be readily available, easily accessed, and financially feasible.

Physical Therapy

Physical therapy plays a major role in the care of persons with MS, especially those with motor, balance, and musculoskeletal difficulties.[1-6] Most physiatrists and physical therapists have considerable experience in treating persons with joint and musculoskeletal injuries, joint surgeries, joint replacements, and arthritis, but the care of persons with MS often requires additional expertise. Persons with MS have significant difficulties with fatigue, heat intolerance, visual and cognitive impairment, and sensory changes, adding to the complexity of their management. Larger physical therapy facilities may have persons experienced in MS care, but smaller facilities may not be able to provide this option. In such instances, referral to a larger facility for initial evaluation and management suggestions, with subsequent transfer of care to a smaller, more convenient facility, may be a reasonable approach.

There are two phases of physical therapy care for persons with MS: during the time of an acute relapse, and during the slowly progressive phase of the disease. During the acute phase of a relapse, disability may peak and then gradually improve. The goal of therapy at this point is to maximize the potential for improvement, with management of joint mobility, balance training, proper use of assistive devices, and strengthening. While admission to the hospital for MS relapses is much less common now than in decades past, admission to an acute neurorehabilitation unit following a functionally impairing attack should be considered. This will allow more intense therapy to be administered and, one hopes, improve outcomes.

Since most physical therapy regimens are approved for weeks rather than months, and improvement after a relapse can continue for up to a year, it is of great importance for therapists to train and motivate both the patient and caregivers to continue as many therapies as possible at home. Periodic follow-up also is important to assess progress, reevaluate and modify the therapy regimen, and continue motivation.[7]

Equally important to the management of persons with MS is physical therapy during the progressive phase of their illness. Neglecting issues such as increasing spasticity and weakness, increasing imbalance, insufficient or incorrect use of assistive devices, joint contractures, and skin breakdown can lead to greatly increased disability, with increased risk for hospitalization, surgeries, and the need for institutional long-term care. Prevention is the best way of avoiding such issues, and periodic physical therapy evaluations and treatments should be available and supported. As noted in Chapter 6, many of the comorbidities associated with MS are the result of increasing disability and lack of mobility. The services of an experienced therapist in mitigating such changes are invaluable.

Physical therapists also can play an important role in the management of bladder and bowel difficulties associated with pelvic floor weakness. Women with MS who have had children may have weakness of the pelvic floor muscles, with increased difficulties with bladder and bowel urgency and control.[8] Instructions in pelvic floor strengthening exercises such as Kegel exercises can significantly help with bladder and bowel symptoms.[9–12]

Exercise Physiologists

The fatigue of MS can be significantly ameliorated by a regular and appropriate exercise program (see Chapter 9). Given the differences in abilities of persons with MS, programs must be individualized to avoid frustration, increased neurologic symptoms, and injuries. The services of an exercise physiologist, experienced in the care of persons with MS, can be of great value, not only in training such individuals but also in providing the motivation necessary for the long-term maintenance of an exercise regimen.

The exercises should be tailored to the abilities and disabilities of the individual. It is beyond the scope of this text to detail specific exercises, but combinations of progressive resistive exercises, passive and assistive range of motion, and aerobic exercises all can have great value.[1,2,4–6,13,14]

Again, there may be two phases in the roles of the exercise physiologist, one during acute relapses and the other during the progressive phase of the disease. Challenges and goals are similar to those noted for physical therapists.

Occupational Therapy

The role of occupational therapists in the care of persons with MS is to allow them to maintain maximal function in the world. Transfers, use of appliances and cars, and modification of devices to allow maximal function are of great value. Energy management and conservation techniques also are important.[15,16] As disease progresses, the homes of many persons with MS become increasingly unsafe and inaccessible. Home assessments and recommendations by occupational therapists are extremely important in terms of allowing an individual with MS to remain at home safely, with minimum hardship for his or her caregivers. Unfortunately, such home assessments are rarely paid for by health insurance, nor is the cost of home modifications. Arrangements with local building supply stores for easement of costs for persons with limited financial resources has been useful in meeting the needs of such individuals.

Psychiatrists, Counselors, and Psychologists

Mood changes, especially depression, anxiety, and stress, are common in persons with MS, especially at the time of diagnosis and as progression of disease necessitates major changes in lifestyle[17–20] (see Chapters 6 and 9). Suicidal ideation is not uncommon, and treatment of such issues requires immediate action by the health professional.[21–23] Because of the stigma of being labeled "crazy," one of the most difficult issues is to persuade individuals that lack of appetite, overeating, irritability and easy angering, insomnia, early morning awakening, hypersomnia, lack of conation, and inability to concentrate and to multitask can all be symptoms of depression. In addition, since a diagnosis of MS and its ramifications can affect family members and caregivers, these individuals' emotional changes also must be addressed. The help of mental health professionals can be of great value in allowing individuals and their families to deal with the changing patterns of MS and to provide critical support during times of greatest stress. Again, choosing counselors and psychologists with knowledge of the disease and its subtleties will greatly increase the value of their counseling and treatment.

Neuropsychologists

Many factors contribute to the cognitive impairment that occurs in many persons with MS, and distinguishing these factors can be difficult with only bedside evaluations. Careful neuropsychometric testing and analyses can help distinguish components of impairment such as depression, fatigue, and intrinsic inabilities due to brain inflammation and loss of tissue. This is done by evaluating the ability to process new information, short- and long-term memory consolidation, executive functions, visual-spatial capabilities, and concentration.

Quantifying cognitive impairment with neuropsychometric testing is also of great value. Such data can help with the management of particular deficiencies, vocational placement, and justification for disability and in more severe cases can support the need for the appointment of conservators or guardians to assist in the management and care of such individuals.

Unfortunately, there is no standard series of neuropsychometric tests for evaluating persons with MS, and great variability exists in the batteries of tests used and their interpretation. Recommendations for test batteries are published,[24–28] and referral to an MS center may provide the best data. Brief testing, such as "mini-mental" tests or the brief tests done by some occupational therapists, are no substitute for the comprehensive information obtained with the extensive evaluations performed by neuropsychologists.

Orthotists

In many persons with MS, orthotics or braces and supports make the difference between ambulation and non-ambulation, between working and loss of employment, and between living independently and needing institutional care.[29–31] The most common orthotics are ankle–foot orthoses (AFOs) designed to treat distal lower extremity weakness and spasticity. Other orthotics, such as knee and hip braces and wrist and finger splints, also allow greater limb function.

In combination with the advice of the physician and the physical and occupational therapists, the expertise of an orthotist is of major value. Compromises in brace design are often needed, with lightness of weight for a weakened limb conflicting with the need for sturdiness and support to control spasticity. Comfort and ease of wear are also essential, with closets of many MS individuals full of devices not worn because of these issues.

Neuro-Ophthalmologists

Persons with double vision and nystagmus can be greatly helped with eyeglass prisms to maintain image convergence. In addition, maximizing visual acuity in persons with optic neuritis is of great benefit, as is determining the presence of non-MS-related causes of visual dysfunction, such as cataracts due to recurrent steroid administration.

Urologists

If decreasing bladder dysfunction occurs that is refractory to the treatments in Chapter 9, a full urologic evaluation is warranted to look for nonneurologic causes of symptoms, such as renal and bladder calculi, cystitis, ureteral or urethral strictures, or hydronephrosis due to chronic urinary retention. Urologists can perform placement and management of suprapubic catheters and can manage male sexual dysfunction with implantation of penile prosthesis and treatment with intracavernous alprostadil.

Social Workers

A social worker with knowledge of long-term care facilities, assisted living facilities, state, county, and city financial support programs, personal and home care attendant options, and the many vagaries of national and private health care insurance can be a great asset in the care of persons with MS. Social workers employed by MS patient advocacy organizations may have particular expertise and resources in meeting the needs of persons with MS.

Diet, Nutrition, and Food Supplements

The cause of MS is not known, but that has not prevented many hypotheses from being promulgated. One of them is that MS, or at least MS symptoms, result from food "allergies" or intolerances. Another is that persons with MS have altered fatty acid metabolism and that intake of saturated fats worsens the disease.

The bottom line regarding the first hypothesis is that there are no persuasive data to suggest that persons with MS have a higher-than-expected incidence of food allergies or food intolerances.[32–34] Obviously, persons with MS who also have gluten intolerance should avoid wheat products, persons with lactose intolerance should avoid milk products, and persons with shellfish intolerance should avoid these foods, but other than such known intolerances, persons with MS do not have special food intolerances.

The other hypothesis suggests that there is an association between intake of saturated fats and the development of MS, that disease is more severe in persons with high saturated fat intake, and that intake of polyunsaturated fats improves the disease (e.g., "Swank diet"). Data in this regard are conflicting, with some small, short-term studies showing a benefit from diets high in omega-3 and omega-6 oils[35] but others showing no benefit.[36] A systematic review in 2007 of all trials involving the effects of diet on the course of MS failed to show any benefits but also found that such diets were safe, with no negative effects.[36] For a variety of other reasons, mainly related to cardiovascular health and obesity, a diet low in saturated fats and high in vegetables, fruits, and salads is to be recommended; this could indirectly help with fatigue and energy improvement. However, there are no data that such a diet has a direct effect on the MS disease process.

The Internet is full of marketers of "food supplements" claiming to have special benefits for persons with MS. Some claim to have "unique water." Others claim that their proprietary vitamins, minerals, and herbs are better absorbed or more complete in meeting the "deficiencies" present in MS, subdue or enhance the activities of the immune system, or can prevent toxicities such as "oxidative stress" or "mitochondrial insufficiencies" that are hypothesized to be associated with the MS disease process. The verbiage accompanying these claims is often extensive, with a scientific veneer that can sound impressive. However, almost all of the evidence offered is either anecdotal or supported by seriously flawed clinical trials. One thing generally true of these purported therapies is that they are much more expensive than standard vitamin and mineral preparations. Herbal products may contain substances of unknown potency, purity, and toxicity. Great caution is advised in the use of unregulated and unproven compounds as either alternative or supplementary treatments for MS.

What is true is that persons with MS should eat a healthy, complete diet, one with sufficient variety to provide all necessary daily nutrients, fluids, and fiber. In persons with or at risk for decreased bone mineral density, supplemental calcium and vitamin D can be recommended. Recent data suggest that lower levels of vitamin D may be associated with an increased risk of developing MS or are a marker for other risk factors.[37,38] Vitamin D plays important roles in immune function,[39] but to date there are no studies supporting a direct therapeutic role for this vitamin in the treatment of MS.

Special diets may be necessary for persons with impaired swallowing or chewing abilities, or those wishing to lose or gain weight, and the expertise of a nutritionist is very valuable for addressing these issues. However, as of this writing, in the absence of established food allergies and intolerances, there is no "special" or "unique" diet or food supplement persuasively shown to affect the disease process in persons with MS.

References

1. Bjarnadottir OH, Konradsdottir AD, Reynisdottir K, Olafsson E. Multiple sclerosis and brief moderate exercise. A randomised study. *Mult Scler*. 2007;13:776–782.

2. Brown TR, Kraft GH. Exercise and rehabilitation for individuals with multiple sclerosis. *Phys Med Rehabil Clin North Am*. 2005;16:513–555.

3. McCullagh R, Fitzgerald AP, Murphy RP, Cooke G. Long-term benefits of exercising on quality of life and fatigue in multiple sclerosis patients with mild disability: a pilot study. *Clin Rehabil*. 2008;22:206–214.

4. Petajan JH, Gappmaier E, White AT, et al. Impact of aerobic training on fitness and quality of life in multiple sclerosis. *Ann Neurol*. 1996;39:432–441.

5. Taylor NF, Dodd KJ, Prasad D, Denisenko S. Progressive resistance exercise for people with multiple sclerosis. *Disabil Rehabil*. 2006;28:1119–1126.

6. White LJ, Dressendorfer RH. Exercise and multiple sclerosis. *Sports Med*. 2004;34:1077–1100.

7. Rasova K, Havrdova E, Brandejsky P, et al. Comparison of the influence of different rehabilitation programmes on clinical, spirometric and spiroergometric parameters in patients with multiple sclerosis. *Mult Scler*. 2006;12:227–234.

8. Wiesel PH, Norton C, Glickman S, Kamm MA. Pathophysiology and management of bowel dysfunction in multiple sclerosis. *Eur J Gastroenterol Hepatol*. 2001;13:441–448.

9. De Ridder D, Vermeulen C, Ketelaer P, et al. Pelvic floor rehabilitation in multiple sclerosis. *Acta Neurol Belg*. 1999;99:61–64.

10. Jameson JS, Rogers J, Chia YW, et al. Pelvic floor function in multiple sclerosis. *Gut*. 1994;35:388–390.

11. McClurg D, Ashe RG, Marshall K, Lowe-Strong AS. Comparison of pelvic floor muscle training, electromyography biofeedback, and neuromuscular electrical stimulation for bladder dysfunction in people with multiple sclerosis: a randomized pilot study. *Neurourol Urodyn*. 2006;25:337–348.

12. Vahtera T, Haaranen M, Viramo-Koskela AL, Ruutiainen J. Pelvic floor rehabilitation is effective in patients with multiple sclerosis. *Clin Rehabil*. 1997;11:211–219.

13. Dalgas U, Stenager E, Ingemann-Hansen T. Multiple sclerosis and physical exercise: recommendations for the application of resistance, endurance and combined training. *Mult Scler*. 2008;14:35–53.

14. Gallien P, Nicolas B, Robineau S, et al. Physical training and multiple sclerosis. *Ann Readapt Med Phys*. 2007;50:369–376.

15. Mathiowetz VG, Finlayson ML, Matuska KM, et al. Randomized controlled trial of an energy conservation course for persons with multiple sclerosis. *Mult Scler*. 2005;11:592–601.

16. Rosenberg JH, Shafor R. Fatigue in multiple sclerosis: a rational approach to evaluation and treatment. *Curr Neurol Neurosci Rep*. 2005;5:140–146.

17. Beiske AG, Svensson E, Sandanger I, et al. Depression and anxiety amongst multiple sclerosis patients. *Eur J Neurol*. 2008;15:239–245.

18. Chwastiak LA, Ehde DM. Psychiatric issues in multiple sclerosis. *Psychiatr Clin North Am*. 2007;30:803–817.

19. Chwastiak LA, Gibbons LE, Ehde DM, et al. Fatigue and psychiatric illness in a large community sample of persons with multiple sclerosis. *J Psychosom Res*. 2005;59:291–298.

20. Korostil M, Feinstein A. Anxiety disorders and their clinical correlates in multiple sclerosis patients. *Mult Scler*. 2007;13:67–72.

21. Feinstein A. An examination of suicidal intent in patients with multiple sclerosis. *Neurology*. 2002;59:674–678.

22. Turner AP, Williams RM, Bowen JD, et al. Suicidal ideation in multiple sclerosis. *Arch Phys Med Rehabil*. 2006;87:1073–1078.

23. Wallin MT, Wilken JA, Turner AP, et al. Depression and multiple sclerosis: Review of a lethal combination. *J Rehabil Res Dev*. 2006;43:45–62.

24. Benedict RH, Fischer JS, Archibald CJ, et al. Minimal neuropsychological assessment of MS patients: a consensus approach. *Clin Neuropsychol*. 2002;16:381–397.

25. Benedict RH, Zivadinov R. Reliability and validity of neuropsychological screening and assessment strategies in MS. *J Neurol*. 2007;254(Suppl 2):II22–II25.

26. Riazi A, Hobart JC, Lamping DL, et al. Evidence-based measurement in multiple sclerosis: the psychometric properties of the physical and psychological dimensions of three quality of life rating scales. *Mult Scler*. 2003;9:411–419.

27. Beatty WW, Monson N. Problem solving by patients with multiple sclerosis: comparison of performance on the Wisconsin and California Card Sorting Tests. *J Int Neuropsychol Soc*. 1996;2:134–140.

28. Bobholz JA, Rao SM. Cognitive dysfunction in multiple sclerosis: a review of recent developments. *Curr Opin Neurol*. 2003;16:283–288.

29. Cattaneo D, Marazzini F, Crippa A, Cardini R. Do static or dynamic AFOs improve balance? *Clin Rehabil*. 2002;16:894–899.

30. DeLisa JA, Hammond MC, Mikulic MA, Miller RM. Multiple sclerosis: Part I. Common physical disabilities and rehabilitation. *Am Fam Physician.* 1985;32:157–163.

31. Ramdharry GM, Marsden JF, Day BL, Thompson AJ. De-stabilizing and training effects of foot orthoses in multiple sclerosis. *Mult Scler.* 2006;12:219–226.

32. Marrie RA. Environmental risk factors in multiple sclerosis aetiology. *Lancet Neurol.* 2004;3:709–718.

33. Payne A. Nutrition and diet in the clinical management of multiple sclerosis. *J Hum Nutr Diet.* 2001;14:349–357.

34. Schwarz S, Leweling H. Multiple sclerosis and nutrition. *Mult Scler.* 2005;11:24–32.

35. Harbige LS, Sharief MK. Polyunsaturated fatty acids in the pathogenesis and treatment of multiple sclerosis. *Br J Nutr.* 2007;98(Suppl 1):S46–53.

36. Farinotti M, Simi S, Di Pietrantonj C, et al. Dietary interventions for multiple sclerosis. *Cochrane Database Syst Rev.* 2007:CD004192.

37. Munger KL, Levin LI, Hollis BW, et al. Serum 25-hydroxyvitamin D levels and risk of multiple sclerosis. *JAMA.* 2006;296:2832–2838.

38. Ozgocmen S, Bulut S, Ilhan N, et al. Vitamin D deficiency and reduced bone mineral density in multiple sclerosis: effect of ambulatory status and functional capacity. *J Bone Miner Metab.* 2005;23:309–313.

39. Smolders J, Damoiseaux J, Menheere P, Hupperts R. Vitamin D as an immune modulator in multiple sclerosis, a review. *J Neuroimmunol.* 2008;194:7–17.

Further Reading

Rao SM, Leo GJ, Bernardin L, et al. Cognitive dysfunction in multiple sclerosis. I. Frequency, patterns, and prediction. *Neurology.* 1991;41(5):685–691.

Rao SM, Leo GJ, Ellington L, et al. Cognitive dysfunction in multiple sclerosis. II. Impact on employment and social functioning. *Neurology.* 1991;l41(5):692–696.

Chapter 11

Gender Issues and Special Multiple Sclerosis Populations

Two thirds of persons with relapsing-remitting MS are women. The reasons for this are not known, but almost certainly genetic and hormonal influences are important. This chapter will review some of the data regarding unique aspects of MS in women, men, children and adolescents, and other special populations.

Women

Whether the pathogenesis of MS is different in women than in men is not known. What is known is that hormonal factors and pregnancy can have profound influences on the course of disease.[1] While medications used to treat MS may have an effect in reducing pregnancy rates, MS per se does not affect fertility,[2] and there no data suggesting that in the long term women having children have worse disease that women who do not bear children.[3–5] Thus, pregnancy should not be discouraged in women with MS just on the basis of their diagnosis.

Menses

It is common for women to note changes in MS symptoms before or during menses.[6,7] Most commonly noted are increasing difficulties with fatigue, weakness, concentration, and mood, at times severe enough to mimic acute exacerbations. The worsening symptoms are not the result of increased CNS inflammatory activity but should be considered "pseudo-exacerbations." In addition, in some women beta-interferons affect menstrual cycle regularity and severity and can also affect thyroid function, usually resulting in hyperthyroidism.

Disease-Modifying Therapies and Pregnancy

The beta-interferons are abortifacients, so use should be stopped before a woman attempts to become pregnant, and certainly once she is pregnant. What is not well defined is how long a woman should wait, if at all, after stopping beta-interferon treatment before trying to become pregnant. I usually suggest waiting for one or two menstrual cycles after stopping beta-interferons. Glatiramer acetate is classified as a category B drug (as opposed to the category C or dangerous classification for beta-interferons):

the risks of using this drug during pregnancy have not been definitively established in humans, but no adverse reactions were observed in animal studies. A small study in women continuing to take glatiramer acetate during pregnancy did not show an increased risk of fetal abnormalities or abortions. Some MS neurologists continue treatment with glatiramer acetate during pregnancy,[8] but most suggest stopping glatiramer acetate during pregnancy and then restarting it after delivery.[9]

Pregnancy

Pregnancy has a profound effect on the course of disease. During the second and third trimesters the disease often goes into remission, only to be followed by an increased risk of relapses in the 2 to 6 months after delivery.[3,10] Identifying women who are at risk for postpartum relapses cannot be done with assurance,[10] but a past history of such attacks would suggest a predisposition to such a pattern. Postpartum MRIs of the CNS may also be of value, with women having a burst of either new T2/FLAIR lesions or lesions with contrast enhancement perhaps being at greater risk. Some data suggest that treatment with intravenous IgG may be of benefit, but large controlled trials are lacking in support of this therapy.[11–14]

Postpartum relapses are no different from any other relapses, and their severity and duration are no different from that woman's previous attacks. The frequency of relapses returns to prepregnancy rates after about 3 to 6 months.[10] Treatment of postpartum relapses is the same as for any other attack.

Restarting Disease-Modifying Therapy and the Role of Breastfeeding

If a woman chooses not to breastfeed, disease-modifying therapy can be restarted immediately after delivery. If a woman chooses to breastfeed, the issue is more complex because the effects of breastfeeding on the course of postpartum MS are not clear. Some data suggest that breastfeeding may be protective and decrease the relapse risk, but the benefits are modest at best.[15] Certainly, breastfeeding does not increase the risk of postpartum relapses. Thus, choosing to breastfeed or not remains a personal choice that could be influenced by the prepartum course of that individual and her perceived need to restart disease-modifying therapy quickly. Finding many new lesions on a post-partum CNS MRI may help in assessing the relapse risk and the need to restart disease-modifying therapy more expeditiously.

There are no data on the consequences of restarting disease-modifying therapy and continuing to breastfeed. As expected, there are differences among neurologists. Most do not recommend restarting disease-modifying therapy during breastfeeding; in those who do restart such therapy, most do so with glatiramer acetate. How long women can "safely" continue to breastfeed in the absence of disease-modifying therapy is also an unresolved issue. The clinical course and MRI changes can be useful in this regard: women with recurrent attacks and those with continuing new MRI lesions may wish to shorten the duration of nursing.

Table 11.1 summarizes unique features of MS in women.

Table 11.1 Unique Features of MS in Women

Feature	Effects on MS	Therapies
Menses	Worsening of MS symptoms, especially fatigue, weakness, imbalance, and emotional lability, usually before but also during menses	• Ensure there are no endocrine or metabolic abnormalities, such as thyroid dysfunction or iron deficiency anemia. • ASA, 650 mg twice a day, is reported to relieve the pseudo-exacerbations of menses. • Birth control pills can modulate the severity of symptoms. If this is not sufficient, the use of long-acting menstrual suppressants can be considered, such as medroxyprogesterone acetate.
Pregnancy	Decreased disease activity during the second and third trimesters, with increased risk of relapses during the 2 to 6 months postpartum	• Consider stopping disease-modifying therapy for one or two menstrual cycles before attempting to become pregnant, especially for women taking beta-interferons. • Relapses occurring after 20 weeks of gestation can be treated with steroids, but caution and consultation with an obstetrician/gynecologist should be considered if treatment is needed at an earlier gestational time. • If the woman chooses not to breastfeed, restart disease-modifying therapy after pregnancy. • In women with a history of postpartum relapses, administration of IV IgG may have preventive value.[11–14]
Breastfeeding	No effect or only a very modest effect in reducing the risk of postpartum relapses	• If the woman is breastfeeding, delay restarting disease-modifying therapy until after nursing unless there is a history of postpartum relapses. If relapses occur postpartum or if postpartum CNS MRIs show increased disease activity, stop nursing, treat relapses, and consider shortening the duration of breastfeeding so that disease-modifying therapy can be restarted.

Men

There are no particular aspects of MS in men that are unique to that gender. Rather, there are differences in the ways that men with MS cope with their illness and in the ways male caregivers are able to accept their tasks. Men may have more difficulty adapting to the diagnosis of MS than women, given their societal roles of "breadwinners" and "protectors" of the family and, compared to women, their relative lack of support networks.[16] Studies

Table 11.2 Pediatric Relapsing-Remitting MS

Category	Characteristic of Pediatric MS	Difference From Adult MS
Age of onset and gender	From early childhood to age 16. In early pediatric MS cases, males and females are almost equal. Female preponderance is noted in postpubertal children with MS.	By definition, age of onset before age 16. Major female preponderance in adult relapsing-remitting MS.
Differential diagnosis	Most importantly, must be distinguished from acute, monophasic CNS inflammatory illnesses such as acute disseminated encephalomyelitis (ADEM). Other illnesses to be considered are neurogenetic metabolic white matter diseases such as adrenoleukodystrophy (ALD), infections such as subacute sclerosing panencephalitis (SSPE), neoplasias, toxic leukoencephalopathies, and vasculitis.[20,21] The most common differential involves distinguishing MS from ADEM. Alterations in levels of consciousness are much more characteristic of ADEM, and recurrences can occur within 3 months of presentation.[22] Recurrent episodes after 3 months are more suggestive of MS.	While there is overlap in the differential diagnosis of the two populations, ADEM is unusual in adults, as are ALD and SSPE.
MRI findings	There are no uniquely different findings from those of adult MS, but there is a tendency for fewer lesions in general, fewer lesions with contrast enhancement, and more posterior fossa lesions.[23] In children under 10, lesions may not meet adult criteria, with ill-defined lesions, involving deep gray matter nuclei too. Lesions of ADEM may not be distinguishable from those of a first attack of MS. As needed for adult MS, new MRI lesions must be separated by an interval of at least 3 months to establish dissemination in time.	No unique features of adult MS MRI changes compared to those of pediatric MS
Clinical course	In general, the course of MS may be slower in pediatric MS, but since age of onset is earlier too, disabilities accumulate at an earlier age. Duration of relapses is less in pediatric MS than in adult MS. However, in children under 10 the course of disease may be more aggressive, with multiple symptoms at onset and with significant residua.[24]	No unique features of clinical course compared to adults
Treatment	• Acute relapses are treated in a similar fashion to adult acute relapses, but dosages must be adjusted. A recommended dosage is 20 to 30 mg/kg/day of methylprednisolone, administered IV over 1 to 2 hour for 3 to 5 consecutive days.[25] Steroid use should be restricted as much as possible in preadolescent children to minimize effects on bone growth.	• Dosages are lower than those used in adults and consequences are different in terms of growth retardation. Otherwise, side effects are similar.

Table 11.2 (continued)		
Category	Characteristic of Pediatric MS	Difference From Adult MS
	• Long-term immune-modulating therapy is similar in pediatric MS to adult MS, but experience with long-term use is limited. Dosages of beta-interferons may need to be reduced for children under age 10, with very gradual dose escalations. Flu-like symptoms can be ameliorated with acetaminophen (15 mg/kg) or ibuprofen (10 mg/kg) at the time of injections and 4 to 6 hours thereafter if needed. No dosage modifications are needed with use of glatiramer acetate.	• Toxicities with beta-interferons, mainly affecting liver, blood count, and thyroid, are similar to adults with MS, and careful monitoring of these functions should be done as in adults, initially monthly for 6 months and then every 3 to 6 months.
	• Criteria for insufficient responders are similar to those of adults and treatments too are similar, but dosages may need to be adjusted. Referral to a pediatric MS center would be appropriate.	• More powerful immune suppressants have been used in adults not responding to usual disease-modifying therapies. These drugs— azathioprine, mitoxantrone, cyclophosphamide, and ethotrexate— have considerable toxicities and their use in pediatric MS should be considered experimental. They should be administered at an MS specialty center.
	• Symptomatic management of pediatric MS is very similar to that of adults with MS. Again, dosages may need to be adjusted.	• Side effects of drugs used for symptomatic management are similar to those seen in adults.
CSF	Frequencies of increased B-cell activation in the form of oligoclonal bands and increased IgG index are similar to those seen in adult MS.	
Psychosocial aspects	Children with MS can have significant cognitive impairment, and this, in association with the emotional difficulties associated with having a chronic disease and their emotional immaturity, makes the management of this patient population especially difficult.[26,27]	Similar emotional and cognitive changes can occur in adults with MS, but there are more defined ways of addressing these issues in adults.

of men as caregivers of spouses also showed that they have more difficulties adapting to that role than women, suggesting that in such situations additional support and assistance for both the patient and the caregiver may be needed.[17,18]

Children of Parents With MS

As is the case with many chronic diseases, MS is an illness that can have profound effects on all family members. Children with parents who have MS may have a particularly difficult time in dealing with this illness, given their relative vulnerability and their inability to understand what may be happening to their parent. Daughters are able to deal with MS in a parent better than sons; sons have even more difficulty dealing with the issues of MS in a father.[19] There are resources, albeit limited, available for children with parents who have MS, and addressing the needs of this population can significantly benefit both the person with MS and his or her children.

Pediatric MS

Pediatric MS is rare, affecting only 2% to 5% of persons with MS, but this population has a different differential diagnosis and different treatment and psychological issues than adults with MS. Pediatric MS occurs in children who are prepubertal, up to the age of 16. While the differential diagnostic possibilities are different than in adults with MS, the criteria for diagnosing the disease are the same—that is, one has to establish the presence of a multifocal, inflammatory CNS disease, affecting predominantly white matter, most often with a relapsing-remitting course, not explained by other illnesses. Table 11.2 details the differences and similarities between pediatric and adult MS.

References

1. Voskuhl RR. Gender issues and multiple sclerosis. *Curr Neurol Neurosci Rep.* 2002;2:277–286.

2. Giesser BS. Gender issues in multiple sclerosis. *Neurologist.* 2002;8:351–356.

3. Damek DM, Shuster EA. Pregnancy and multiple sclerosis. *Mayo Clin Proc.* 1997;72:977–989.

4. Houtchens MK. Pregnancy and multiple sclerosis. *Semin Neurol.* 2007;27:434–441.

5. Runmarker B, Andersen O. Pregnancy is associated with a lower risk of onset and a better prognosis in multiple sclerosis. *Brain.* 1995;118(Pt 1):253–261.

6. Wingerchuk DM, Rodriguez M. Premenstrual multiple sclerosis pseudo-exacerbations: Role of body temperature and prevention with aspirin. *Arch Neurol.* 2006;63:1005–1008.

7. Zorgdrager A, De Keyser J. Menstrually related worsening of symptoms in multiple sclerosis. *J Neurol Sci.* 1997;149:95–97.

8. Coyle PK, Christie S, Fodor P, et al. Multiple sclerosis gender issues: clinical practices of women neurologists. *Mult Scler*. 2004;10:582–588.

9. Ferrero S, Esposito F, Pretta S, Ragni N. Fetal risks related to the treatment of multiple sclerosis during pregnancy and breastfeeding. *Expert Rev Neurother*. 2006;6:1823–1831.

10. Vukusic S, Hutchinson M, Hours M, et al. Pregnancy and multiple sclerosis (the PRIMS study): clinical predictors of post-partum relapse. *Brain*. 2004;127:1353–1360.

11. Achiron A, Kishner I, Dolev M, et al. Effect of intravenous immunoglobulin treatment on pregnancy and postpartum-related relapses in multiple sclerosis. *J Neurol*. 2004;251:1133–1137.

12. Durelli L, Ricci A, Verdun E. Immunoglobulin treatment of multiple sclerosis: future prospects. *Neurol Sci*. 2003;24(Suppl 4):S234–238.

13. Haas J. High-dose IVIG in the post partum period for prevention of exacerbations in MS. *Mult Scler*. 2000;6(Suppl 2):S18–20; discussion S33.

14. Haas J, Hommes OR. A dose comparison study of IVIG in postpartum relapsing-remitting multiple sclerosis. *Mult Scler*. 2007;13:900–908.

15. Nelson LM, Franklin GM, Jones MC. Risk of multiple sclerosis exacerbation during pregnancy and breast-feeding. *JAMA*. 1988;259:3441–3443.

16. Miller A, Dishon S. Health-related quality of life in multiple sclerosis: The impact of disability, gender and employment status. *Qual Life Res*. 2006;15:259–271.

17. Good DM, Bower DA, Einsporn RL. Social support: gender differences in multiple sclerosis spousal caregivers. *J Neurosci Nurs*. 1995;27:305–311.

18. Anderson ML. Daring men to be caring men: the dilemma of disability for male caregivers. *Axone*. 2001;22:18–21.

19. Steck B, Amsler F, Kappos L, Burgin D. Gender-specific differences in the process of coping in families with a parent affected by a chronic somatic disease (e.g. multiple sclerosis). *Psychopathology*. 2001;34:236–244.

20. Banwell B, Ghezzi A, Bar-Or A, et al. Multiple sclerosis in children: clinical diagnosis, therapeutic strategies, and future directions. *Lancet Neurol*. 2007;6:887–902.

21. Hahn JS, Pohl D, Rensel M, Rao S. Differential diagnosis and evaluation in pediatric multiple sclerosis. *Neurology*. 2007;68:S13–22.

22. Tenembaum S, Chitnis T, Ness J, Hahn JS. Acute disseminated encephalomyelitis. *Neurology*. 2007;68:S23–36.

23. Banwell B, Shroff M, Ness JM, et al. MRI features of pediatric multiple sclerosis. *Neurology*. 2007;68:S46–53.

24. Ness JM, Chabas D, Sadovnick AD, et al. Clinical features of children and adolescents with multiple sclerosis. *Neurology*. 2007;68:S37–45.

25. Pohl D, Waubant E, Banwell B, et al. Treatment of pediatric multiple sclerosis and variants. *Neurology*. 2007;68:S54–65.

26. MacAllister WS, Boyd JR, Holland NJ, et al. The psychosocial consequences of pediatric multiple sclerosis. *Neurology*. 2007;68:S66–69.

27. MacAllister WS, Christodoulou C, Milazzo M, Krupp LB. Longitudinal neuropsychological assessment in pediatric multiple sclerosis. *Dev Neuropsychol*. 2007;32:625–644.

Chapter 12

Resources

Web Sites

- Consortium of MS Centers: http://www.mscare.org/cmsc/index.php
- National Institute of Neurological Disorders and Stroke—MS Information Page: http://www.ninds.nih.gov/disorders/multiple_sclerosis/multiple_sclerosis.htm
- Listing of pediatric MS centers: http://www.nationalmssociety.org/about-multiple-sclerosis/who-gets-ms/pediatric-ms/pediatric-ms-centers-of-excellence/index.aspx

Patient Advocacy Organizations

- National Multiple Sclerosis Society: http://www.nationalmssociety.org/index.aspx
- Multiple Sclerosis Association: http://www.msassociation.org/
- Multiple Sclerosis Foundation: http://www.msfocus.org/
- Paralyzed Veterans Association: http://www.pva.org/site/PageServer

Sites for Disease-Modifying Therapies

- http://www.avonex.com/msavProject/avonex.portal
- http://www.betaseron.com/
- http://www.copaxone.com/
- http://www.mslifelines.com/rebif/index.jsp
- http://www.tysabri.com/tysbProject/tysb.portal
- http://www.rxlist.com/cgi/generic/mitoxantrone.htm

Site for MR Imaging Protocol for MS

- http://www.mscare.org/cmsc/Vancouver-2003-Guidelines-for-a-standardized-MRI-protocol-for-MS.html

Patient Books and Materials

Many of the patient advocacy organizations noted above have large numbers of books, pamphlets, and videos available for persons with MS and their families. A publisher that specializes in books on MS is Demos Medical Publishing: http://www.demosmedpub.com/.

Index

Notes